D0430568

VITAMIN C: THE MASTER NUTRIENT

VITAMIN C

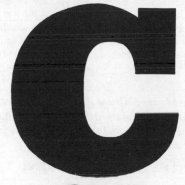

The Master Nutrient

Sandra Goodman, Ph.D.

Foreword by Richard A. Passwater, Ph.D.

Keats Publishing, Inc. ✦ New Canaan, Connecticut

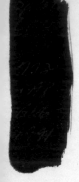

ACKNOWLEDGEMENTS

Sincerest appreciation and gratitude for the vision and optimism of George Klabin and for personal and technical support from Mike Howell. I write this book as a contribution toward the development of an integrated and holistic paradigm of health care which will embrace and work on all levels—body, spirit and psyche—of the individual in need.

Vitamin C: The Master Nutrient is not intended as medical advice. Its intent is solely informational and educational. Please consult a health professional should the need for one be indicated.

VITAMIN C: THE MASTER NUTRIENT

Copyright © 1991 by Sandra Goodman, Ph.D.

All Rights Reserved

No part of this book may be reproduced in any form without the written consent of the publisher.

Library of Congress Cataloging-in-Publication Data

Goodman, Sandra
   Vitamin C, the master nutrient / Sandra Goodman.
     p.   cm.
   Includes bibliographical references and index.
   ISBN 0-87983-571-0 : $9.95
   1. Vitamin C—Popular works.   2. Vitamin C—Therapeutic use.
I. Title.
QP772.A8G66   1991
612.3'99—dc20   90-23227
                                            CIP

Printed in the United States of America

Published by Keats Publishing, Inc.
27 Pine Street (Box 876)
New Canaan, Connecticut 06840-0876

CONTENTS

Contents

Preface

WHAT'S DIFFERENT ABOUT THIS BOOK

What will you learn from this book about vitamin C that you have not already read or heard about from the plethora of excellent books and journal articles already on the market or in the scientific literature? A perfectly valid question for the discerning nutritionally conscious consumer or health practitioner.

One of the main themes which will be emphasized in this book is that in addition to being a vitamin, which by definition is required for life in tiny amounts, vitamin C, or ascorbic acid, is actually an essential nutrient, which, taken in optimal quantities, can vastly improve health and prevent many serious conditions, including heart disease, diabetes, and cancer. Even a fairly superficial review of what has been written about vitamin C reveals perhaps hundreds of books and thousands or even ten thousand research papers on the subject. There have been three entire

Vitamin C: The Master Nutrient

conferences of the New York Academy of Sciences devoted to vitamin C alone over the past two decades! Linus Pauling, dual Nobel prize winner (Chemistry 1954, Peace 1962) and eminent scientist and statesman, has rigorously and eloquently put forward the attributes of vitamin C with more than 500 references appended in his book *How to Live Longer and Feel Better* (Avon, 1986). Dedicated and erudite experts Irwin Stone, Emanuel Cheraskin, Ewan Cameron, Marshall Ringsdorf, and Emily Sisley, to name but a few, have authored books and performed clinical studies which have put vitamin C on the map and before the public eye more than any other nutritional supplement[1,30,35,43,50,54,164,166,200].

And, although a fascinating historical saga of great importance, the nutritionally informed reader probably does not need to be reminded at length of how in 1747 the British naval physician James Lind experimentally discovered a preventive for scurvy in citrus fruits, which is at the origin of the inaccurate term "limeys" later attributed to British sailors. This book, written in light of and with respect to the immense body of knowledge which has been established historically about vitamin C, is a present– and future-oriented look at the exciting developments taking place which will certainly alter our views about fundamental biochemical workings of the body.

So what else, the reader may ask, is there to say about this vitamin which has been touted as a miraculous cure for just about everything from the common cold to hemorrhoids? And who is this person who purports to add another volume to the already heavy vitamin C bookshelf?

What's Different About This Book?

This book:

1. Critically analyzes the most up-to-date scientific information about vitamin C, especially pertaining to its therapeutic efficacy and mode of action with respect to illnesses including atherosclerosis, diabetes, rheumatoid arthritis and cancer;

2. Presents for the first time ever in popular print, rigorous and astonishingly encouraging laboratory results detailing vitamin C's antiviral activity against the Human Immunodeficiency Virus (HIV);

3. Describes for the first time in book form, the development of a novel form of vitamin C, trade name Ester-C ascorbate, and presents clinical data and critical analyses to document and explain aspects of its apparently superior mode of action.

As for my position, I am a scientist by training and profession. In addition to my role as a Health Consultant, I am also, as are we all, a consumer of health care. I find myself, at this point in history, situated in two worlds virtually at war with each other, although each speaks sincerely of its commitment to the well-being of its patients. I speak of course of the medical and scientific "establishment" on the one hand, and the naturopathic, alternative or complementary practitioners on the other. Having been trained both in orthodox and alternative practices, I understand and empathize with how this tremendous schism came into being between these two "solitudes." I also grieve for the sick individual who is suffering and who is entitled to the best that all traditions can offer. I'm one of many who are committed and are working toward constructing a tangible bridge to connect these two worlds with the goal of developing an improved paradigm of health care that will embrace the best of Western technological medicine with the efficacy and safety of traditional natural medicine.

Vitamin C is both an outstanding example as well as a victim of this rather disharmonious situation. Reams of literature abound attesting to the clinically therapeutic and preventive value of this nutrient; yet probably the majority of medically trained physicians still hold the outdated view that amounts of vitamin C in excess of that sufficient to prevent scurvy are a waste of money and simply produce "expensive urine." Linus Pauling has documented numerous examples of misinterpreted, badly designed and/or poorly executed clinical trials purporting to "objectively" investigate the efficacy of vitamin C and has eloquently painted the dismally divided research scenario[116]. Pity that despite disparagement of the reputation of such an eminent scientist, many physicians do admit, off the record, that vitamin C works.

For, despite the voluminous legacy of words and data which already exists regarding vitamin C, there is breakthrough and exciting new information which has only recently been discovered, and which must be told. New information which has only very recently been released within the scientific world is starting to shed light on vitamin C's ability to be a potent force in the fight against AIDS, heart disease, diabetes and to counter the free-radical pathology involved with rheumatoid diseases. In addition, the commercial development of a new form of vitamin C called *Ester-C ascorbate,* which contains extra natural metabolites, has serendipitously thrust the limelight further into the biochemical mechanisms behind the action of vitamin C.

What's Different About This Book?

This book brings together the latest research being performed on many aspects of vitamin C's therapeutic action. This information, properly implemented, may save countless lives and promote better health. And, in interpreting some of the facets which appear to enhance the action of vitamin C and Ester-C ascorbate (which, interesting enough, have a connection with the latest vitamin C/AIDS research), the gap between the research scientist, physician and the lay person can be bridged, facilitating an improvement in health care.

I have not spent decades devoted to vitamin C research, as have Linus Pauling and dedicated others. I do not own nor do I have any interests in the sales or promotion of vitamin C or, for that matter, of any other commodity. Nor do I purport to have all the answers which will magically settle the controversy which presently pits much of the medical and scientific establishment against nutritionally oriented practitioners. Nevertheless, the application of a scientific as well as a holistic approach to the subject of vitamin C and health can be an invaluable contribution to that day when many more illnesses will be prevented, and when the majority of illnesses can be healed using more refined, and less harmful therapeutic practices than at present.

This book cannot even attempt to review all the existing literature about vitamin C. This book starts out by bringing you up to date with a short historical retrospective about vitamin C. After summarizing some of vitamin C's fundamental health-empowering roles including immune enhancer and free radical scavenger, this book brings you the most up-to-date information, gleaned from many and varied sources, about how vitamin C can help in treatment for diabetes, heart disease, cancer and rheumatoid arthritis. Then, this book is the first to describe the elegant experiments which demonstrate the power of vitamin C against the AIDS virus, and attempts to interpret how this action may be happening. Next comes the exciting story of the development of Ester-C ascorbate, whose properties enable it to be more efficiently absorbed and retained than other forms of vitamin C. Finally, this book addresses you, the consumer, and fields questions each individual will encounter in forming his or her own decision about whether to take vitamin C, which form, and how much.

For it is you, the individual person who must ultimately decide how much vitamin C to take—whether your glass of orange juice will also contain several or many grams of vitamin C, whether it will be ascorbic acid, one of the ascorbates, or the new Ester-C ascorbate. In any case, a toast to your health, and enjoyable reading.

Foreword

Richard A. Passwater, Ph.D.

The scientific excitement continues about the vitamin C family of nutrients. Our knowledge of the
health roles that the vitamin C family play continue
to grow daily as scientific study after scientific study
reveals more about them until at last it has become
apparent that vitamin C is the "Master Nutrient."

The vitamin C family includes vitamin C, vitamin
C metabolites, and the vitamin C "helpmates,"—the
bioflavonoids. Vitamin C activity is provided by ascorbic acid, mineral ascorbates, and other ascorbate
compounds.

Scientists have long been aware of the importance
of bioflavonoids, as at one time they were even
thought to be vitamins themselves. At first, Nobel
Prize winner Dr. Albert Szent-Györgyi called the bioflavonoids "vitamin P." Now we recognize that bioflavonoids are semi-essential secondary food factors.

Vitamin C: The Master Nutrient

But recent research with formerly little-known bio-flavonoids such as pycnogenol and quercitin is causing scientists to look afresh at the earlier importance of the bioflavonoids as envisioned by Dr. Szent-Gyorgi.

Vitamin C: The Master Nutrient may be the first book to describe in detail the research of vitamin C along with its natural metabolites of the aldonic acid family. These metabolites are proving to have unexpected and exciting results that potentiate vitamin C and increase its effectiveness. The most important metabolites, L-threonic acid, L-xylonic acid and L-lyxonic acid appear to aid in the retention and circulation of active vitamin C, and even help transport vitamin C into both fat-based and water-based systems. Dr. Sandra Goodman states that the discovery of the modulating roles of metabolites will almost certainly rewrite all our textbooks to make room for the treatment of vitamin C's many physiological and hormonal roles in the body.

Dr. Sandra Goodman also breaks new ground with details on the research of Dr. R. J. Jariwalla at the Linus Pauling Institute on how vitamin C inhibits HIV reverse transcriptase activity and thus inactivates the AIDS virus. The far-reaching implications of the research of Dr. Anthony Verlangieri of the University of Mississippi's Atherosclerosis Research Laboratory is also reviewed. Dr. Verlangieri has shown that added vitamin C to the diet reduces deposits in the arteries.

These aforementioned are only two of the many areas in which vitamin C works. Dr. Goodman describes a significant portion of the known area of vitamin activity, and the reader will come to understand why vitamin C is being called "The Master Nutrient."

Vitamin C: The Master Nutrient has substance to offer to both the health professional and the lay person. Both need to understand the broad base of vitamin C activity and be updated on the new research presented. This is must reading as no health professional is fully informed without the knowledge of vitamin C presented here. In fact, all of us are responsible for our own health and for being fully informed about this "Master Nutrient."

Introduction

VITAMIN C—PAST, PRESENT AND FUTURE

To put this saga in proper perspective, we should begin this tale about 60 million years ago. For that's when, according to biochemist Irwin Stone, our ancestors lost the ability to make their own vitamin C^{200}. But we did NOT lose our requirement for considerable amounts of this life-sustaining and critical nutrient on a daily basis. Our loss of self-sufficiency with respect to vitamin C and our subsequent dependence upon diet to provide adequate amounts has impacted significantly our health and lifestyle throughout history, relevant especially today in our polluted, nutrient depleted, stressful high-tech "advanced" world. We have indeed travelled (fallen) a long way since our proverbial exit from the paradisiacal garden of Eden, where presumably there was an abundance of citrus fruits and vitamin C.

Time warp. Middle Ages. Sailors expiring by droves—exhaustion, depression, muscle pain, haggard appearance, bleeding gums, stinking breath, hemorrhaging and extensive bruising, diarrhea, lung/kidney troubles, death. Scurvy. Dead sailors of all nationalities—Portuguese, Spanish, British, French. Horrible voyages, many corpses and countless unaccomplished missions.

1536. Jacques Cartier, Quebec City, Canada. Iroquois Indian remedy for scurvy—tea made from the leaves and bark of the arbor vitae tree determined centuries later, to possess high vitamin C content.

1747. British physician James Lind performed a now famous clinical trial on twelve of his men suffering from scurvy. He divided the men into six groups, receiving daily, in additional to their normal diets, either: two oranges and one lemon; cider; dilute sulfuric acid; vinegar; sea water; or a mixture of drugs. After six days the men receiving the citrus fruits were well, all ten others remained ill. This and other experiments were later published in Lind's "A Treatise on Scurvy," 1753.

In today's world obsessed with double-blind placebo-controlled trials, Lind's work would have been criticized on the basis of the small sample size, lack of placebo and lack of double blind. The British Admiralty, despite the huge losses incurred from this devastating condition, waited 48 years until 1795 before decreeing that daily rations of fresh lime juice be given to sailors in the British Navy. Although scurvy disappeared very soon thereafter from the British Navy, it continued its scourge throughout the British merchant marine for another 70 years, until the Board of Trade followed suit with a similar decree in 1865.

1911. Theory of "vitamines" published by Polish biochemist Casimir Funk working in London, theorizing that four substances found in natural foods confer protection against the diseases of beriberi, rickets, pellagra and scurvy. In 1913 the American E.V. McCollum started the modern nomenclature system of vitamins, by referring to "fat-soluble A," "water-soluble B," scurvy-preventing "water-soluble C" and rickets-preventing "fat-soluble D."

1928. First isolation of pure vitamin C by Hungarian biochemist Albert Szent-Györgyi working in Cambridge England, the Mayo Clinic, Minnesota and Hungary[202]. Szent-Györgyi isolated a substance which he named hexuronic acid, and which was subsequently shown, in 1932, to be vitamin C by American scientists Waugh and King[233]. Typical of so many scientific discoveries, Szent-Györgyi was not actually searching for vitamin C. He was attempting to identify an oxygen-combining substance which prevents the appearance of brown pigment from decaying fruit. His diverse expertise in oxidation-reaction and physiology enabled him to isolate a large enough quantity of hexuronic acid from cabbages, adrenal glands of animals, as well as that favorite Hungarian spice, paprika. Following the determination by Szent-Györgyi of the substance's chemical formula $C_6H_8O_6$, and the determination of its structural formula in collaboration with the English chemist Haworth, the chemical name for vitamin C was changed from hexuronic to ascorbic acid, denoting an acidic substance which prevents and cures scurvy.

Research directed at the determination of the level of vitamin C necessary to prevent scurvy led to the establishment of a recommended dietary allowance (RDA) for vitamin C of 60 mg per day[179]. And, basically, what most scientists and doctors are taught

3

in their medical training about nutrition is that certain nutrients prevent certain deficiency diseases. There is abundant evidence that this minimal RDA-level of 60 mg in no way reflects the optimal level of vitamin C required for excellent health. In fact, Irwin Stone blames the emphasis of vitamin C as an antiscurvy vitamin rather than an essential nutrient since the 1930s for halting progress of clinical research and therapeutic application of vitamin C for the treatment of a wide number of diseases. During the 1940s and '50s, Dr. F.R. Klenner pioneered large doses of vitamin C for the treatment of many viral diseases, including poliomyelitis[126-8].

We of the late twentieth century are so smug. The word scurvy induces an almost knee-jerk smirk and the thought "oh, scurvy doesn't exist anymore—a glass of orange juice, vitamin C, etc." Scurvy is a boring subject which has been relegated to the annals of history and such for school-aged children. Well, look again at the symptoms and forget the name of the disease: exhaustion, depression, muscle pain, haggard appearance, bleeding gums, stinking breath, hemorrhaging and extensive bruising, diarrhea, lung and kidney troubles. Who amongst the most fit and active super specimens has not occasionally experienced degrees of several or all of the above symptoms? Perhaps we have been so clever in categorizing every substance into a pigeon-hole in relation to a given disease that we have totally ignored the universal and massively complex biochemical roles played by substances such as vitamin C.

The American biochemist Dr. Irwin Stone published in 1965 an evolutionary treatise expounding that by a chance genetic mutation in the required vitamin C enzyme machinery, humans and several other animal species lost their ability to make vitamin[199]. The time estimates for this genetic event vary from between 25 to 60 million years. According to this theory, because we lack the crucial vitamin C manufacturing ability, humans generally suffer from a genetic disease called hypoascorbemia (deficiency of ascorbic acid), which in mild form produces chronic health problems such as high cholesterol, heart disease, arthritis, colds and cancer, and in severe cases leads to the fatal condition of scurvy.

As a theoretical framework, the concept of a flexible continuum of vitamin C required for optimal health is impeccable, especially when integrated with each person's biochemical individuality, environmental and nutritional history and lifestyle and stress factors.

In 1970 Linus Pauling produced shock waves throughout the medical establishment by publishing his first book *Vitamin C, the Common Cold and the Flu*[164] in which he documented evidence of vitamin C's efficacy, and presented extensively researched, sometimes searing yet well-deserved critiques of scientific investigations and trials previously conducted, some of which arrived at erroneous conclusions or seriously understated or omitted their positive findings from abstract summaries of their studies.

Throughout the 1970s research burgeoned investigating vitamin C's interactions with the immune system, therapeutic action in the treatment of postoperative patients, cancer, heart disease, diabetes, while in the marketplace different forms of vitamin C appeared: mineral ascorbates, buffered and time-released capsules.

5

Vitamin C: The Master Nutrient

1981. In his landmark paper "Vitamin C, Titrating to Bowel Tolerance, Anascorbemia, and Acute Induced Scurvy"[46], Dr. Robert Cathcart described a method to determine one's optimal level of ascorbic acid and revealed the successful use of ascorbic acid in treating over 9,000 patients with conditions including mononucleosis, hepatitis, bacterial infections, allergy, Candida albicans, trauma, surgery, burns, cancer, disc-related back pain, arthritis, scarlet fever, herpes and populations with high frequency of crib death. In 1984 Dr. Cathcart published another paper[47] describing the use of vitamin C in the treatment of AIDS. As the 1980s progressed, so did the research, clinical and consumer use of versatile vitamin C increase astronomically. Linus Pauling published his bestseller *How to Live Longer and Feel Better*[166] in 1986, with meticulous research and references summarizing therapeutic uses of vitamin C; likewise Drs. Cheraskin, Ringsdorf, and Sisley in *The Vitamin C Connection—Getting Well and Staying Well With Vitamin C*[54]. The New York Academy of Sciences' Third Conference on vitamin C was held on July 7, 1987[36], bringing together scientific papers about vitamin C in subjects such as neurochemistry, epidemiology, biochemistry and immunology, diseases such as diabetes, cataracts and eye disease, free radicals, and metabolic requirements and safety.

During the 1980s a tiny fledgling company, Oxycal Laboratories Inc. in Prescott, Arizona, while researching a novel ascorbate production process, determined that natural byproducts, called metabolites, in their vitamin C product greatly enhanced its absorption and retention. Ewan Cameron and Linus Pauling, in their book *Cancer and Vitamin C*[43], farsightedly pre-

6

dicted that "these oxidation products (metabolites), which as yet have not been thoroughly studied, may provide an important part of the mechanism by which large doses of vitamin C help to control cancer and other diseases." United States Patent No. 4,822,816 was assigned to Oxycal Laboratories for this improved form of Vitamin C, trade-named Ester-C ascorbate, on April 18, 1989[146].

At the 2nd International AIDS Symposium in Feb. 1989 in Los Angeles, Dr. Raxit Jariwalla, Director of the Immune Deficiency and Viral Carcinogenesis Department of the Linus Pauling Institute presented a paper documenting that vitamin C was capable of inhibiting, by 99 percent, the reverse transcriptase (RT) activity of the AIDS virus in laboratory cells infected with the Human Immunodeficiency Virus (HIV)[97]. Molecular biology experiments suggest that byproducts or metabolites of vitamin C may be responsible for this anti-HIV activity.

The future with respect to vitamin C is really only beginning. The biochemistry of the metabolism of vitamin C in the body is only crudely understood. The role of metabolites, the subject of exciting research into atherosclerosis and diabetes, may reveal aspects of vitamin C not even thought of several years ago. And still the controversial debates rage among all the experts in this "respectable" yet contentious field: whether vitamin C causes kidney stones or alleviates kidney stones; the advisability of taking massive doses versus the requirement to take massive doses to experience benefit. The experts argue over the best composition of vitamin C—ascorbic acid, buffered ascorbates, Ester C, and in what form—crystals, tablets, capsules or intravenous injections.

7

Vitamin C: The Master Nutrient

The saying goes that "wherever there is smoke, there is fire." Well, the corollary to this truism must be "wherever there is fire there is inspiration." So, to you, the reader, whether practitioner, researcher or health-minded consumer, sit back and enjoy the substance and the fireworks of the vitamin C debate, remembering that you are the final arbiter of your health and health care, and that no "expert" is omniscient.

Chapter 1

VITAMIN C: THE DIFFERENCE BETWEEN SICKNESS AND OPTIMAL HEALTH

Health is emphatically not merely the absence of disease. Just because we are not suffering from hay fever, runny nose, arthritis, cancer, heart disease, or stomach upset, does not mean that we are at the peak of health. However, being free from all physical illness would certainly be an excellent start on the journey to total health. And we are the best judges of our own state of health. Can you remember a time when you felt absolutely fit, completely relaxed and sublimely interested and motivated and enamored with every aspect of your life? This uncommonly experienced state in today's world probably describes what optimal health is about.

Just as every individual is endowed with a unique set of genes, has a unique history of physical, biochemical, nutritional and emotional experiences, so the measure of optimal health is probably unique for each of us. Optimal mean "the best we can be." The number of "minor" health problems plaguing the average individual is amazing—allergies, stiffness, back pain, hemorrhoids, skin rashes, fatigue, headache. We have become so used to these "minor" complaints that we only use the term illness to describe the even more serious problems which follow as we overload our body's capacity to handle abuse—arthritis, heart disease, diabetes, cancer.

Can you imagine that you could be free from health complaints and therefore ready to devote your energies to really living your life fully? It is possible, and accomplishing this will probably take you into vistas hitherto untravelled. You may discover and correct food allergies that are contributing to your minor health problems, dietary and environmental pollutants that contribute to illness and lifestyle practices which relax you and help you to more effectively manage your daily stress.

Vitamin C, nutrient extraordinary, has been shown to be one of the body's vital substances required for many fundamental processes, ranging from the biosynthesis of collagen, fat-transporting carnitine, the hormones adrenaline and cortisone, electron transporter in many enzymatic reactions, protector of the integrity of blood vessels, promoter of healthy gums, radiation protector-regulator of cholesterol levels, free radical detoxifier, antibacterial and antiviral agent and immune enhancer.

The use of vitamin C within your health program will certainly augment your state of health and may significantly treat and prevent many serious illnesses. Vitamin C, along with other health-promoting substances, may enable you to experience, perhaps for the first time in a long time, the radiant feeling of optimal health, as opposed to the sub-optimal absence of overt disease.

Therapeutic Uses of Vitamin C

The following is a list of many of the conditions for which preventive application or treatment with vitamin C has been shown to be effective:

AIDS

Alcoholism and drug addiction

Allergies, food and environmental

Anxiety, stress

Asthma

Atherosclerosis (hardening of the arteries)

Bed sores

Bacterial infections

Burns

Cancer (bladder, breast, bronchial, cervical, kidney, liver, lung, ovarian, rectal, skin)

Candida albicans infections

Colds

Depression

Diabetes

Glaucoma

Heart disease

Hemorrhoids

Hepatitis

High cholesterol

Influenza

Chronic fatigue syndrome

Mental illness

Mononucleosis

Pain

Periodontal disease

Postsurgical trauma
Radiation damage
Rheumatoid arthritis, rheumatoid diseases
Rhinitis (hay fever)
Sudden Infant Death Syndrome (as a preventive)
Ulcers
Viral infections
Wounds and physical trauma

What Is Optimal Health?

This indeed is one of the most intelligent and important questions at the center of our growing renaissance in understanding optimal health and well-being of the individual and our entire society. The answer, simple, yet the subject of voluminous scientific, philosophical and spiritual treatises throughout the millennia, is that optimal health is embodied by balance amongst all levels of ourselves—physical, emotional, mental and spiritual. Illness or dis-ease (lack of ease or disharmony), is the result of imbalance. We are not compartmentalized automatons—we are intricately connected and exquisitely orchestrated organisms, sensitive and responsive to all that we take into our bodies, minds and psyches.

Vitamin C is an integral substance required for the normal functioning of our bodies. Since so many of us are unbalanced by virtue of deficient diet, environmental toxins and lifestyle stresses, is it not therefore reasonable that restoring adequate amounts of a fundamentally essential nutrient can help to restore health, whether the physical location of the disease be the eyes or the feet or the heart?

The scientific and technological advances of the past several centuries, along with the widespread adoption of a rational, scientific and mechanistic world-view have engendered the almost universally accepted notion that one disease = one cause = one cure.

And certainly, since the discovery of bacteria and the concomitant development of many disease-specific drugs such as antibiotics, most people assume that there is a specific cause and cure for each disease. Hence the long, expensive and as yet unsuccessful search for "magic bullets" for multifactorially-caused diseases such as rheumatoid arthritis, cancer and heart disease. And witness the arousal of our skepticism and accusations of quackery when claims are made for natural products which apparently can cure or alleviate everything from hay fever to housemaid's knee.

If Vitamin C Is So Good, Why Doesn't My Doctor Prescribe It?

Hopefully in the near future, many more physicians will be prescribing vitamin C and other natural health promoting substances. Much of the clinical research reported upon in the massive vitamin C literature originates from physician-directed case histories and trials. Hopefully as well, the stereotyped images of pill-pushing G.P.s, knife-obsessed surgeons and radiation and chemotherapy-oriented cancer specialists, will make way for a more interdisciplinary and humane, and less invasive, model of health care. Ask ten different specialist practitioners, ranging from G.P. to acupuncturist, to suggest treatment for an individual with certain ailments, and almost certainly there will be a diversity of opinion, just as asking ten economists or politicians for their suggestions for a given economic or political situation may produce ten radically different policies.

Is it heresy to expose the truth that doctors, like the rest of humanity are not omniscient, and do not have the "secret" knowledge to make you better? Within each healing speciality, a competent practitioner should be able to prescribe treatment, drugs, potions, that work for a particular illness. Each specialist will, of course, be influenced by their particular type of training. The surgeon is more familiar with surgery and would not ordinarily recommend nutritional supplements for a heart condition. The orthomolecular physician might recommend chelation therapy rather than a triple bypass operation for someone with atherosclerosis. It would be most unusual for a radiologist to recommend Chinese herbs for treatment of a tumor, or a Chinese doctor to prescribe homeopathic medicines for a cancer patient, etc. Yet all these disciplines, including stress management and counselling, might be valuable and appropriate in treating each of these conditions.

The cooperation of a wide spectrum of practitioners, including orthodox and "complementary" nourishing of the mind as well as the body of the patient, will end the current polarized situation which sees battles rage between medical associations and just about every other discipline. Moreover, the impetus to bring about such an improved situation may rest with health-conscious consumers who must learn to assert themselves when it comes to choosing health-care options. Consumers have learned admirably to consult with friends and competitors in choosing houses, cars, stereos, holidays; similarly, the individual should take individual responsibility for what happens to his or her body.

This means asking the practitioner about treatment options, possible side effects from suggested treatment, and making a considered decision about what to do on the basis of thorough research of the possible consequences. The practice of putting oneself in the hands of one's doctor and leaving it up to him or her should be adopted only after researching the options and deciding upon the chosen course of treatment. We are all in the driver's seat when it comes to our health. The doctor and every other practitioner is merely here to assist us in our recovery. The consumer must stop playing the role of passive recipient and assume a more active and responsible approach to health care.

Can Vitamin C Actually Cure All These Illnesses?

This is what each of us who is actually suffering from one of the above conditions secretly wants to know: Is vitamin C the "magic bullet" for each of us? We are gradually finding out that we are our own healers. Ultimately, it is we who, with the aid of food, potions, drugs, laughter, and any number of other methods, get better. However, along the road to optimal health, the truth is that vitamin C is an excellent companion, having been shown to be a most effective, and totally safe health promoting substance for each of the above listed conditions.

This book makes no claim that vitamin C alone, or for that matter, anything else alone, will prevent or cure the above conditions. Life and health are too complex and dependent upon too many variables to guarantee such a sweeping and naive claim. However, epidemiological and clinical data show very strong correlations between vitamin C intake and levels and incidence of many illnesses. And clinical trials and treatment of tens of thousands of patients with vitamin C over several decades provide us with a solid foundation of therapeutic evidence.

The development of Ester-C ascorbate and the discovery of the utility of metabolites have catapulted us into a new level of enquiry that may assist in unravelling the biochemical workings of this amazing vitamin. This book will attempt to explain the mechanisms behind vitamin C's versatile therapeutic successes. Within the following pages is the clinical research evidence describing vitamin C's effectiveness with many of the major scourges of our age— cancer, heart disease, diabetes, rheumatoid arthritis, AIDS and chronic fatigue syndrome.

Chapter 2

MYTHS AND FACTS

Rumors, Claims and Fantasy

Which expert can you believe, especially when they are all so sincere? How can you know which "facts" to believe, which to question and which to dismiss as errant nonsense? These are far from trivial issues, especially in a saga as complex, long-standing and contradictory as that related to vitamin C. Although it's not uncommon to have a majority of "experts" in any given scientific field at loggerheads and in intense competition with each other, it is not an everyday occurrence that a major scientific figure of a century with two Nobel prizes has to almost single-handedly "take on" the scientific and medical establishment in order to convince them of a substance's therapeutic efficacy. That Linus Pauling has to a large degree achieved this goal, in that the medical evidence in favor of vitamin C's health-enhancing

17

properties is now overwhelming, is a tremendous testimonial of this man's foresight, tenacity and scientific wizardry.

However, what's the public to think when prominent and respected researchers disagree and contradict each other? Whom can you believe and trust? Unfortunately, you have no choice but to exercise some human qualities like skepticism, discrimination and good old-fashioned common sense. This is actually what scientists are taught during their career, to always be critical, to always keep an open mind and to never get attached to the absolute truth of any theory. A safe bet is to regard the "truth" as the "best working hypothesis" of the day.

There is a fair degree of criticism of the scientific and medical research establishment throughout this book, especially regarding the slow pace and minimal level of funding of research related to natural substances such as vitamin C compared to more expensive and toxic drugs. Be that as it may, there is still much to be said for the elaborateness of procedures of the scientific method, where eventually facts get unearthed and distinguished from erroneous hypotheses, conjectures and premises.

This is not, however, the case for articles appearing in the various media (newspapers, magazines, newsletters), which, not subjected to the rigid constraints of the scientific community, can run riot in sensationalism, panic mongering and elaborate fantasy, with the apparently well-intentioned motive of exposing dangerous facts. Below are several quotations from one such article[22], extremely convincingly written, and with interesting and speculative hypotheses and theoretical conclusions presented as irrefutable facts.

The author alleges that vitamin C may be responsible for causing: infection, gum problems, depression, exhaustion, personality changes, blood sugar problems, and many other things, including cancer.

You could take every book on vitamin C and throw it in the East River! You'll probably be a lot healthier for it.

Vitamin C is lost from the body so readily because it causes dramatic physiological effects that could be dangerous.

The inability to produce vitamin C internally may be one of the greatest things that has elevated human beings over animals. Vitamin C reduces copper levels, and the absence of internally produced ascorbic acid may have allowed a higher level of copper to exist in human brains. There is one species of dog, the Bedlington Terrier, who has extremely high levels of copper and who is so intelligent that some owners consider it to be "almost human."

This confirms my suspicion that in some people—about 10-20 percent of the population, excess vitamin C can contribute to bone problems such as osteoporosis.

I know from my own experience that C supplements over 500 mg a day cause me extreme fatigue. I have also talked to two other people who had similar results.

Rather than literature citations, the author, a "publisher," speaks of his opinion, his suspicion, his experience. He cites no research, merely speaking of his own subjective opinions, or that of several friends. It's outrageous that such serious, unsubstantiated allegations can be published; consider the potential harm such alarmist fantasy could do, while raising fears in the public. While personal experience is always to be valued, the discriminating consumer bears in mind that his own experience is as valid as the next, and that neither may represent the whole situation. Articles such as this are exceedingly provocative and as such are valuable in enabling us to look at the facts and our beliefs in a critical light; however, if the allegations are mistaken, unsubstantiated and believed by an uncritical reader, there is no scientific organization to which the author can be held accountable. No self-respecting scientist would dare to make such sweeping prognostications about complex physiological phenomena. Hence the eternally appropriate "caveat emptor"—buyer beware— for each of us.

Over the years vitamin C has been implicated in causing certain conditions and interfering with certain diagnostic tests[99]. These issues have recently been thoroughly reviewed by Cheraskin[54] and Pauling[166]. An updated summary of the major concerns and latest evidence is presented here.

Myth: Vitamin C Causes Kidney Stones. As indicated in Fig. 3, oxalic acid is one of the byproducts of vitamin C metabolism, and there has been a rather long-standing concern that consumption of large amounts of Vitamin C could cause the formation of calcium oxalate kidney stones. The clinical evidence[132,212-3]

20

recently reviewed separately by Cheraskin[54], Pauling[166], and Rivers[178] indicates that in fact, vitamin C does not cause kidney stones in "normal" individuals[188]. The several reported such cases involving vitamin C indicate that oxalate metabolism and contributory factors to kidney stones are rather complicated: other factors include dietary oxalate consumption, low calcium and magnesium intake, EDTA consumption, B6 deficiency, high tryptophan, vitamin D and sucrose, low water consumption and persistently acid urine.

In fact, some research indicates that oxalate may actually be a minor component in kidney stone formation, in that some people with normal oxalate excretion make kidney stones, and others with large oxalate excretion do not[54]. According to Rivers at the Third International Conference on Vitamin C in 1987, "ingestion of large quantities of the vitamin (C) does not constitute a risk factor for calcium oxalate stone formation in most healthy persons."

Cheraskin[54] and Cathcart[49] have both pondered why vitamin C does not seem to produce kidney stones, even though oxalate metabolism can be increased. Both these physicians, with clinical experience with many thousands of patients, have reached similar theoretical conclusions about why vitamin C may actually prevent kidney stones:

1. Vitamin C makes the urine more acidic, thereby reducing the binding of calcium with oxalate;

2. Vitamin C binds calcium, thereby reducing calcium's free form, making it unavailable for binding with oxalate;

3. Vitamin C enhances the frequency of urination, making it less likely for stones to form;

4. Vitamin C is a mild urinary tract disinfectant, thereby reducing the foci of infections around which calcium oxalate crystals could be deposited.

There do appear to be individuals who may have a congenital defect in their oxalate metabolism and who are therefore prone to forming kidney stones. Since calcium oxalate stones form in acidic urine, using forms of vitamin C which keep urine alkaline such as sodium ascorbate may prevent these stones[166]. Individuals with such a history or tendency should explore vitamin C, and indeed, their entire supplementation program, with a professional orthomolecular physician. Individuals with a history of kidney stones, renal impairment and individuals on kidney dialysis should not ingest large amounts of vitamin C unless under medical supervision[178]. Further clinical research documenting the effects of the different forms of vitamin C, including the mineral ascorbates and Ester-C ascorbate, would help to lay to rest this theoretical concern which has not materialized among the considerable populations of vitamin C users.

Myth: Vitamin C Causes Gouty Arthritis. Concerns that vitamin C could cause gouty arthritis in predisposed persons have not been borne out; not a single report has appeared in the literature[54,166]. In fact, vitamin C has recently been proposed as a treatment for gout, due to its ability, with high doses, to lower serum uric acid levels. According to Rivers, "The evidence does not support claims for an ascorbic acid induced uricosuria"[178].

Myths and Facts

Myth: Vitamin C Destroys Vitamin B. The original report by Herbert & Jacob[102], alleging that vitamin C destroys vitamin B12 has been refuted by several reliable research studies[2,103,144-5,160]. The study by Herbert & Jacob was severely flawed in that it contained errors in estimating the amount of vitamin B12 contained in food by a factor of five. Again, Rivers[178]: "The evidence has consistently demonstrated that vitamin B12 in food and the body is not destroyed by ascorbic acid."

Myth: Vitamin C Causes Sterility. The proposed hypothesis in the mid-1970s that vitamin C might prevent conception and thus reduce fertility in women has not been substantiated, and has been refuted by physicians such as Abram Hoffer[54]. In fact, in experiments carried out in Japan and Ireland[54], it appears that vitamin C may actually increase fertility and aid in conception, in addition to regulating ovulation and controlling spontaneous abortion in pregnant women[166].

On the male side, research indicates that vitamin C may enhance male fertility. A placebo-controlled trial with 30 men conducted by Dawson and coworkers[66] indicated that vitamin C improved sperm in terms of total count, viability, motility and reduced sperm agglutination.

Myth: Vitamin C Causes Iron Overload. Vitamin C is one of the main promoters of dietary iron absorption, along with meat and fish[96]. Vitamin C can form soluble iron complexes and reduce ferric to ferrous iron. The main dietary inhibitors of iron absorption are phytates found in pulses and polyphenols[96]. Tea, and to a lesser extent, coffee, inhibit iron absorption[183]. Vitamin C's enhancement of iron absorption is normally regarded as a positive attribute; nevertheless, concerns have been raised postulating that vitamin C could have the effect of increasing iron absorption so much as to cause excessive iron or iron overload.

According to Rivers, who recently reviewed the research evidence, "the regulatory mechanisms that control body iron stores override any pronounced alterations in food iron availability . . . Concern that massive doses of ascorbic acid might lead to excessive iron, accumulated in healthy iron-replete individuals appears unwarranted"[178].

In fact research indicates that vitamin C can actually help to reduce excessive iron stores in individuals with iron-overload disorders. Such individuals have subnormal white blood cell levels of vitamin C, caused by their excessive iron storage. When Vitamin C is administered to restore normal white cell levels, excessive iron is excreted[231].

Therefore the evidence seems to point to vitamin C having a pivotal homeostatic role with respect to iron—it promotes iron absorption in iron deficient individuals and accelerates iron excretion in people with excessive iron.

Myth: Vitamin C Interferes with Serum Glucose Levels and Causes Diabetes. Concerns that taking high doses of vitamin C could affect serum glucose levels, interfere with diagnostic blood and urinary tests for glucose[148] and actually cause diabetes have prompted studies to assess vitamin C's effect upon blood and urinary glucose levels.

Studies by Katz & Di Silvio[124], Prauer[170], and Spiegel and Pinili[194] clearly showed that serum glucose levels are not affected by vitamin C, and that taking large doses of vitamin C would not interfere with glucose blood tests. In order to determine whether vitamin C could interfere with urinary glucose, especially important for diabetics, Nahata & McLeod[159] performed a total of 360 copper detection tests on ten male subjects' urine samples, with replicates for each of the four dosage regimes, ranging from 4 to 6 gm vitamin C. Not a single false-positive reaction occurred. Tests have also been developed in which vitamin C does not interfere with urinary glucose determinations[34].

Vitamin C Interferes with Urinary Tests and Blood Stool— Yes and No. Jaffe and coworkers at the NIH reported in 1975[114] that ingesting large quantities of vitamin C masks the detection of blood in stool samples, and, in 1979[115], of blood in urine, and for several years it was required to stop vitamin C supplementation for 24 to 36 hours previous to having blood stool and urine tests performed. However, Dr. Jaffe, being a resourceful clinical pathologist in addition to a strong advocate of vitamin C's therapeutic effects, went on to develop a new test for blood in the stool which is not interfered with by vitamin C[116]. However, until such time as a blood in urine detection test is developed which is not masked by vitamin C, it will still be necessary to refrain from taking vitamin C prior to taking such a diagnostic test.

Vitamin C: The Master Nutrient

Myth: Vitamin C Causes Rebound Scurvy. Allegations that suddenly stopping vitamin C after taking prolonged large doses could actually cause "rebound scurvy"[214] have been investigated in research studies. Hornig and co-workers, after administering massive doses of vitamin C to guinea pigs over a prolonged period, reported that results "disprove the hypothesis that the regular ingestion of large doses of ascorbic acid may lead to systemic conditioning, i.e., accelerated ascorbic acid metabolism or excretion due to a possible induction of the participating enzymes"[106].

Nevertheless, it is vital that vitamin C not be stopped suddenly, especially with individuals with cancer and AIDS[43,48,166]. A sudden depletion of that person's ascorbic acid level could massively lower their resistance, making them extremely vulnerable to infection and disease. When large doses of vitamin C are taken, the entire enzymatic machinery, including metabolites, goes into operation[166]. In this way, because of an adequate supply of ascorbic acid, more of vitamin C is converted to metabolite products. If vitamin C is suddenly withdrawn, the person's biochemistry will continue to produce these metabolites for a week or two, despite the fact that there is not an adequate vitamin C level in the blood. Since vitamin C is so vital for almost every body system, from brain to heart to the immune system, this can be exceedingly dangerous for severely ill persons.

For these reasons, it is most important that anyone who has been taking more than 5 g vitamin C daily on a maintenance dosage taper off gradually, if they decide to reduce their daily vitamin C supplementation.

Summary of Vitamin C Safety Considerations

As reported by Rivers in the 1987 Vitamin C Conference[178], "the practice of ingesting large quantities of ascorbic acid will not result in calcium oxalate stones, increased uric acid excretion, impaired vitamin B12 status, iron overload, systemic conditioning or increased mutagenic activity in healthy individuals." In other words, do not necessarily panic when reading alarming articles about the dangers of vitamin C. They may not, and thus far in fact, have not been true. No reported case of a serious illness from vitamin C exists, and in animal studies, administration of 1/2 of a percent body weight of vitamin C produced no side effects. This amount translates into 350 g for a human being!

The Vitamin C Network—Mineral and Drug Interactions

The nature of the interaction of vitamin C with other nutrients—vitamins and minerals, and drugs[176]— is far from completely understood. In the summation report of Rivers at the most recent Vitamin C Conference in 1987[178], "The interaction of ascorbic acid with dietary essential mineral elements other than iron is not included in this review. Research on this topic is revealing interesting results, but is insufficient at this time to formulate valid conclusions."

Although there may not as yet be comprehensive knowledge regarding the interaction of vitamin C and other nutrient elements and drugs, there have been to date, at least preliminary data demonstrating

Vitamin C: The Master Nutrient

some of the complex synergistic actions of vitamin C with other substances. These are summarized in Table 1 below:

Table 1. Interactions of Vitamin C with Other Nutrients

NUTRIENT	VITAMIN C	CO-FACTORS	REF.
Calcium	Assists in calcium absorption	Mg, CT,PTH	93
Cadmium	Reduces body burden of cadmium	Zinc	38,65
Chromium	Alters toxic form of chromium		
Copper	May reduce copper levels		65,168
Cysteine	May reduce levels of cysteine		65
Folic acid	Prevents destruction of folic acid		65
Iron	Enhances absorption of iron		96
L-carnitine	Required for synthesis of L-carnitine		135
Lead	Reduces body burden of lead, copper, zinc		38,65
Lysine	May reduce levels of lysine		65
Mercury	Reduces body burden of mercury		38,65
Zinc	May reduce levels of zinc; is a co-factor of zinc in prostaglandin synthesis		

The above data are to be regarded as preliminary; in fact, an article by Calabrese et al.[38] failed to show any effect at all of vitamin C upon levels of cadmium, lead and mercury in 45 males over a two-month period. However, these individuals had normal levels, and it would be more appropriate to study the effect of vitamin C in individuals with a high body burden of these toxic metals.

28

Vitamin C and Drug Interactions

Just as vitamin C can modulate the action of certain drugs[25,173,192] (see Chapter 11) so can certain drugs affect vitamin C's effects[93,99]. It is emphatically suggested that individuals who are taking such medications become fully informed about the entire range of their side effects and metabolic interactions. A brief compilation of some of the major drugs and their interactions with vitamin C is presented in Table 2:

Table 2. Vitamin C and Drug Interactions

DRUG	IINTERACTION WITH VITAMIN C
Alcohol	Vitamin C detoxifies, prevents "hangover" and liver damage[245]
Aspirin	Depletes vitamin C levels, inhibits vitamin C absorption[54,65]
Anticoagulants	Vitamin C decreases anti-coagulant effects
Barbiturates	Deplete vitamin C levels. Vitamin C increases barbiturate effects[93]
Heroin	Vitamin C relieves withdrawal symptoms[79]
Methadone	Vitamin C relieves withdrawal symptoms[79,187]
Oral contraceptives	Deplete vitamin C levels[54]
Sulfa drugs	Decrease vitamin C effects[93]
Tetracycline	Decreases vitamin C effects[93]
Tobacco	Depletes vitamin C levels[192]. Smokers use 25 mg of vitamin C per cigarette, which translates into ½ g per pack.
Tranquilizers	Vitamin C assists in withdrawal, reduces withdrawal side effects[54]

Vitamin C: The Master Nutrient

Vitamin C, Alcohol Detoxification and Relief of Hangovers

Research investigating vitamin C's ability to aid in detoxification following alcohol and drug abuse is one of the most promising avenues of research being pursued today[54,79,187]. In a highly promising report prepare by Zannoni and co-workers[245] at the Third Conference on Vitamin C, vitamin C was described as being able to oxidize alcohol in the following manner: vitamin C generates a peroxide which is then used by catalase in the oxidation of alcohol. The body has an ascorbate-dependent detoxification system which is more active than the alcohol dehydrogenase or cytochrome P-450 microsomal systems. In one study, whereas half the alcohol-dosed guinea pigs developed liver necrosis, none of the vitamin C-treated animals developed liver damage.

In humans vitamin C was demonstrated to significantly enhance alcohol clearance, and even to effect substantial improvements in behavior, especially motor coordination. And, since vitamin C reduces fat accumulation in the liver following alcohol consumption, it appears that vitamin C may protect against direct damage to the liver from alcohol.

Experiments for the Future

The interaction of vitamin C (itself such a ubiquitous and complexly integral part of the entire body's biochemistry) with other equally complex vitamins and minerals, is not simple. Biochemistry and homeostatic metabolism normally provide for an elaborate system of feedback loops and safety valves, to ensure our proper functioning. Knowledge about how large doses of vitamin C interact with other essential nutrients is eagerly awaited.

Chapter 3

VITAMIN C AND ESTER-C METABOLISM AND METABOLITES

Vitamin C Literacy

Before embarking upon an investigation into the therapeutic powers of vitamin C, a summary of some of the technical language and constituents involved in the formulation of various products is provided which may prove useful to the consumer and professional alike.

Chemical formulae and biochemical pathways are not engraved in stone upon the brains of scientists, at least not upon that of the author. Even after many years and advanced courses in biochemistry, physiology, etc., these pathways fade from memory unless in constant use. And, with the incredibly rapid advances in knowledge occurring in science and medicine, much material may simply be new and not have been taught during one's formal training. These formulae are presented here as aids in understanding as well as a handy reference tool.

A brief synopsis is included here for the layperson; figures and more details appear in the Appendix for health professionals.

Structure and Biosynthesis of Vitamin C

Vitamin C is also known as ascorbic acid. This 6-carbon molecule is structurally very similar to the sugar D-glucose (Fig. 1). This is significant because of the way vitamin C works to fight diabetes and heart disease.

Vitamin C, found naturally throughout most of the plant and animal kingdom, is synthesized from glucuronic or galactonic acid derived from the sugar glucose in the biosynthetic process shown in Fig. 2.

Humans, non-human primates, guinea pigs, the red-vented bulbul (an Asian bird), the Indian fruit-eating bat, rainbow trout and Coho salmon are the only animal species lacking the complete enzymatic machinery to synthesize vitamin C. It has been shown that humans and guinea pigs lack the enzyme gulono-lactone oxidase, which oxidizes 1-gulonolactone to 2-keto-1-gulonolactone. This, then is the 25 to 60 million-year-old evolutionary accident spoken of earlier which has deprived humans and these other animals of their ability to synthesize their own vitamin C. Whether, as genetic engineering techniques become more refined in the future, it may become feasible to reintroduce this enzyme back into human cells, must remain a subject beyond the scope of this book, however fascinating an idea it may be.

Vitamin C: The Master Nutrient

Ascorbate salts

Preparations of vitamin C are frequently obtainable as salts of ascorbic acid, commonly as sodium or calcium ascorbate. Sodium (calcium) ascorbate is prepared from ascorbic acid and sodium (calcium) carbonate by controlled precipitation in dilute acetone or alcohol[184]. Ester-C ascorbate, prepared totally in aqueous solutions, has not, therefore, been exposed to these toxic chemicals. The more neutral pH and buffering power of ascorbate salts compared with ascorbic acid is frequently cited as a superior attribute of ascorbate products.

Metabolites.

These may be the magic potentizers in vitamin C research today and in the near future. Metabolites are substances or constituents that form part or take part in the metabolism of a substance. Other possible terms are *by-products* or *chemical intermediates,* i.e., intermediate products in vitamin C metabolism. Although vitamin C research has been going on for over four decades, we are still at the infant stage in really unraveling exactly how vitamin C gets absorbed and metabolized at the cellular level. The study of vitamin C's metabolites may be crucial to shedding light on some of these crucial biochemical questions, which may lead to profound and perhaps powerful breakthroughs in several areas of medical science. The metabolism of vitamin C into its constituent metabolites is shown in Figure 3 in the Appendix.

Ester-C Ascorbate

The form of vitamin C sold under the trade name Ester-C refers to a composition of vitamin C, normally an ascorbate salt, which also contains at least one of vitamin C's naturally-occurring metabolites. The manufacturing process of Ester-C ascorbate is unique in that all reactions are carried out with aqueous solutions (water) and there is no use of organic solvents (acetone, alcohol) as in previous methods of ascorbate precipitation. The presence of metabolites in Ester-C in significant quantities accounts for superior absorption and retention properties compared to ascorbic acid and ascorbates[229].

Chapter 4

VITAMIN C—THE IMMUNE EMPOWERER

Many serious and debilitating illnesses arise from malfunctions in the competence of the immune system. Such disorders include AIDS and other immunodeficiency conditions such as chronic fatigue syndrome, as well as conditions resulting from the immune system attacking its own cells (autoimmune disease), such as arthritis. The importance of an optimally functioning immune system is highlighted by what happens when the immune system is deliberately suppressed, such as when organ transplant operations (heart, bone marrow, etc.) are performed. Although it's necessary in such instances to suppress the immune response to prevent rejection of the transplanted organ, the individual is left extremely vulnerable to infection even from normally innocuous agents. The most dramatic illustration of the importance of the immune system occurs when a child is born with a defective immune system, and must live in a "plastic bubble" in order to protect against opportunistic infection.

With the advent of AIDS and the increased incidence of other immune-related conditions (including allergies) during the last decade, we have all become fairly well-informed about the immune system—that "defense network" of specialized and intricately coordinated cells which are charged with the task of maintaining our bodies free from foreign invaders: lymphocytes, antibodies, T-cells, killer cells, macrophages, interferon.

The study of immunology has of late become intertwined with neurochemistry and psychology, forming a field called psychoneuroimmunology, which is almost breathtakingly complex and intricate in its design and function. Not only does the body have several different types of defenses against foreign attack (cell-mediated, humoral, complement), but within each of these different systems is a considerable variety of different components and chemical substances, each forming a finely tuned and coordinated cascade of biochemical events.

The immune system is comprehensive with components residing within each cell, as well as specially organized centers, including the lymph nodes, throughout the body. However, notwithstanding the voluminous scientific information which has accumulated on many aspects of the immune system, we are still somewhat in the dark about how to optimally empower our immune system so that we remain in the best of health.

The truth is that health, and its opposite side of the coin, illness, is a complexly-determined entity, involving many factors—hereditary genetic makeup, nutritional history during pregnancy and early infancy, the geographical region where we live, environmental contaminations and pollution, our psychological and emotional makeup, our lifestyle, the amount of stress and how we handle it, our eating habits, abusive behavior (including smoking, drinking and overeating foods like sugar and animal fats).

The equation for health is a uniquely determined formula for each person. However, just as a universal formula that will work for everyone, cannot be devised, there is a considerable body of evidence which demonstrates that there are a number of nutritional compounds, including vitamin C, which can help strengthen the immune system, reduce free radical formation and thereby, in combination with good eating habits, sensible lifestyle and proper stress management, promote optimal health.

The Vitamin C–Immune Connection

1. Leukocytes require vitamin C for effective function. A landmark discovery, once again the result of serendipity, is that vitamin C is required for proper leucocyte function[6]. Leukocytes are the body's white blood cells, a vital component of the immune system. Researchers investigating leukocytes from guinea pigs, realized that the unusually fragile leukocytes were the result of vitamin C deficiency[30]. The scorbutic (suffering from scurvy) guinea pigs' leukocytes were so depleted of vitamin C that they could not reject tissue transplants. Upon supplementation with vitamin C, the leukocytes functioned normally, and the guinea pigs were able to reject the skin grafts[166].

Lymphocytes, a phagocytic (cell-devouring) type of leucocyte, are particularly important to immune responses in cancer and only function effectively as phagocytes if concentrations of vitamin C are high[108]. In an experiment to test the relationship between vitamin C and reproduction of lymphoctyes, Yonemoto at the National Cancer Institute demonstrated a direct relationship between levels of vitamin C supplementation and the budding of new lymphocyte cells (blastogenesis)[242]. Five grams of vitamin C doubled the rate of lymphocyte budding, 10 g vitamin C trebled the rate, and 18 g quadrupled the rate of lymphocyte blastogenesis! Who knows? The optimal rate of vitamin C for lymphocyte blastogenesis may exceed 18 g in individuals such as cancer patients, whose lymphocytes are severely depleted of vitamin C.

Vitamin C, in addition to modulating the new production of lymphocytes, is also crucial to their rapid mobilization to the site of infection, and their effective phagocytic activity. A multitude of factors, including colds, cigarette smoking and stress, severely deplete the vitamin C levels from leukocytes, rendering the individual more vulnerable to secondary infection. A study by Hume and Weyers (1973)[111] determined that 1 g vitamin C per day plus 6 g per day at the onset of a cold, kept the leukocytes operationally effective in their phagocytic "clean-up" activity.

2. Vitamin C modulates antibody levels. Antibodies are one of the immune system's most direct lines of defense against infectious foreign substances or antigens. When the body is exposed to such an organism, or compound, clones of antibodies are produced against the antigen, which attack and destroy it. There are a variety of classes of antibody molecules, with corresponding different functions within the complex immune system. Levels of three of these classes of antibody molecules—IgA, IgG and IgM—have been found to increase with increased vitamin C levels. As can be seen from Table 3, IgA, IgG and IgM are involved with the body's defenses against bacteria and other microbes, viruses, foreign particles and pathogenic substances.

In a study conducted by Vallance of British subjects isolated for a year in Antarctica[217], it was found that antibodies IgG and IgM increased with increased

Table 3. Types of Antibodies

ANTIBODY FUNCTION

IgA Concentrates in body fluids (tears, saliva, respiratory, genitourinary and gastrointestinal secretions) guarding body entrances. First line of defense against invading pathogens and food allergens. Major Ig in defense against viruses.

IgD Major Ig present on surface of B cells; may be involved in differentiation of these cells.

IgE Involved in allergic reactions. Attaches to surface of mast cell and on encountering its matching antigen stimulates the mast cell to pour out its contents. Also fights parasites.

IgG Most common. Major Ig in defense against microbes. Coats microorganisms, speeding their destruction by other immune system cells. Confers long-standing immunity.

IgM Major Ig produced in primary antibody response. Circulates in the bloodstream where it kills bacteria. Increases during acute stage of an infection. Usually forms in star-shaped clusters.

From *Maximum Immunity*, M.A. Weiner, 1986. Gateway Books.

vitamin C intake. Similarly, in a placebo-controlled study conducted by Prinz and colleagues[171], it was found that 1 g vitamin C per day resulted in significant increases in serum levels of IgA, IgG and IgM. Similar correlations with vitamin C and antibody levels have also been found in guinea pigs, which, like man, cannot synthesize their own vitamin C, and must rely upon external sources for this vital nutrient.

3. Vitamin C modulates synthesis of complement. Complement is a non-cellular immune component which is composed of a complex cascade of 20 enzymatic proteins which can modulate antibody-antigen reaction. Vitamin C is involved in the synthesis of the Cl-esterase component of complement, and levels of this efficacious compound increase with increased vitamin C intake[166].

4. Vitamin C modulates interferon synthesis. Interferons (there are as many as 20 different types) are proteins with antiviral activity, produced in cells which have been infected with virus, and also possibly in malignant cells. Interferon is being experimentally tested in treatment of different forms of cancer; however treatment with externally synthesized interferon rather than with the body's own naturally produced interferon, may have toxic side effects. Recent evidence confirms that increased vitamin C intake results in increased interferon levels[208]. Thus, vitamin C is a "natural" antiviral treatment[62].

5. Vitamin C modulates prostaglandin synthesis. The prostaglandins are a class of small lipid molecules which, acting as hormones, play a role in blood flow heartbeat regulation, cell damage by drugs and immune response. Two prostaglandins in particular, PGE2 and PGF2, are involved in tissue inflammation causing swelling, pain, tenderness and heat. Vitamin C has been shown to inhibit the synthesis of PGE2 and PGF2-alpha, thus exerting an anti-inflammatory effect. The prostaglandin PGE1 modulates lymphocyte formation, thus playing a key role in immune response. Vitamin C increases the synthesis of PGE1[109], thus, in yet another way, contributing to the optimal functioning of the immune system.

With even this brief look at vitamin C's interactions with the immune system, it can be readily appreciated that vitamin C levels are intimately linked with immune function. The level of vitamin C in an individual can make the difference between a weak, barely adequate, or a strong immune response to infection and illness. Since the very cells of the immune system require adequate levels of vitamin C to function effectively in their activities, it's clear that vitamin C can be a most powerful ally in the quest for optimal health.

Chapter 5

VITAMIN C SCAVENGES POISONOUS FREE RADICALS

It is astonishing how long the list has become of substances toxic to health. Even apart from the environmentally derived poisons including lead from auto emissions, pesticides, nitrates, ozone, radioactive exposure, mercury from dental fillings, PCBs, etc., it is also true that many natural processes and substances vital to life and health can also do us in. Including, amazingly, oxygen, the breath of life.

In the words of Etsuo Niki, contributing scientist from the University of Tokyo at the New York Academy of Science Conference on Vitamin C[161], "Oxygen is a double-edged sword. We cannot live without oxygen, but at the same time we are continuously exposed to oxygen toxicity. The free radical-mediated peroxidation of biological molecules and tissues has received much attention in connection with a variety of pathological events such as heart disease, rheumatoid arthritis, inflammatory disorders, cancer and even the aging process." This is the introduction to Niki's research paper describing the synergistic action of vitamins C and E in combating toxic oxygen species.

What then are free radicals and toxic oxygen species? Why are they so dangerous? And what is vitamin C's role in neutralizing and destroying these toxic species?

Free radical oxygen species, some of which are toxic, are highly reactive, unstable molecules because they have lost an electron. Examples include hydrogen peroxide, superoxide, hydroxyl radical and singlet oxygen. In the chemical drive to replace that missing electron, free radicals may initiate an entire cascade of chemical reactions, resulting in damage to membranes, DNA mutations, accelerated ageing, disruptions in cell vitality and function, and deposition of fat. Reactant oxidant species are thought to underlie the cause of many diseases; the use of natural antioxidants is widely advocated in the treatment and detoxification from such conditions[101].

Contrary to what one might think, free radicals are not always externally derived; they occur and are generated in the body's natural biochemical course of living and metabolism, through the oxidation of polyunsaturated fats, the increased generation of adrenalin and noradrenalin under stress, and even as toxic weapons used by phagocytes, some of the foot soldiers of the immune system. External sources of free radicals include exposure to low levels of nuclear radiation and electromagnetic emissions, smog with its powerful oxidants such as ozone, nitrogen dioxide, and peroxyacyl nitrates, cigarette smoke, and environmental pollutant drugs and chemicals[65].

Reassuringly, however, there are a number of natural substances, including vitamin C, which are powerful antioxidants and free radical scavengers, and which act to prevent the damaging effects of superoxides, peroxides, hydroxyl radicals and singlet oxygen molecules. These include the preventive antioxidants catalase and peroxidase and chain-breaking antioxidants which scavenge radicals to stop free-radical and chain-propagation reactions. The water-soluble, chain-breaking antioxidants include vitamin C, uric acid, cysteine and glutathione, while the lipid soluble antioxidants such as vitamin E function within membranes. A list of toxic oxidants and some of their known respective scavengers is presented in Table 6 in the Appendix. It's highly likely that many more such natural scavengers exist in nature, awaiting our discovery.

Vitamin C scavenges superoxide and hydroxyl radical[182], as well as reacting directly with hydrogen peroxide, therefore protecting against various toxic free radicals which promote lipid peroxidation[33]. For example, the generation of toxic oxygen species by phagocytes is associated with a number of chronic degenerative and inflammatory conditions, including cancer, arthritis and lung disease. Laboratory experiments have demonstrated that vitamin C neutralizes these harmful oxidants derived from phagocytes[7]. Vitamin C after being converted to dehydroascorbic acid by free radical reactions, is regenerated via the glutathione enzyme complex[161]. It is interesting that the vitamin C (ascorbate) free radical itself, rather

45

than initiating radical chain reactions, does not react with oxygen and quenches itself very rapidly. And since vitamin C reacts directly with hydrogen peroxide, it acts as a protectant against damage from lipid peroxides.

However, an even more fascinating chapter in the vitamin C-free radical protection story is the finding that vitamin C and vitamin E work together, synergistically, in inhibiting the free radical chain oxidation of lipids[161]. Vitamin C actually regenerates the vitamin E radical, enabling these two potent antioxidants to cooperate in what is called redox coupling.

It had been noted previously that vitamin C "spared" the consumption of vitamin E in free radical chain oxidation experiments; however, it had never been shown whether vitamin C, located in the aqueous part of the cell, and vitamin E, situated within the lipid membrane, could actually cooperate to prevent these detrimental lipid peroxidation events. Results reported on at the latest Vitamin C Conference showed that, in fact, even though vitamin C is sequestered in the aqueous part of the cell and cannot penetrate the lipid membrane, that vitamin C is accessible to the vitamin E radical and does regenerate vitamin E[161]. Since Ester-C ascorbate is fat soluble, its vitamin E regeneration activity may be superior to that of vitamin C.

Multiple sources of free radicals abound: chemicals in our food; heating unsaturated oils, margarine and other unsaturated fats[74-5]; not to speak of the toxic chemicals ingested from pesticides, nitrites, etc. In the face of this growing menace from so many seemingly unavoidable threats to our health, there would appear to be two typical "knee-jerk" reactions for the individual:

1) To scrupulously avoid contact with every conceivable toxic substance, environment, food and stress, since stress plays a major role in releasing free radicals; or

2) To throw up one's hands in despair and do nothing, deciding that it's not possible to eliminate toxins from life in the twentieth century.

The first response, taken to extremes, could lead to an acutely neurotic and/or hermetic lifestyle (taking to the clean air of the Himalayas to meditate alone for the rest of one's life); the second, likewise could provide an excuse or rationalization for laziness in controlling one's daily living habits.

What then, is a sensible response to this ever-mounting barrage to our health from so many sources? Is there something we can do in the face of so many health threats around every corner? It makes sense to inform ourselves thoroughly and accurately about health risk factors such as free radicals and toxic oxygen species without going overboard in panic, and to implement as many health promoting measures in our lives as feels appropriate and convenient. Obviously there are degrees of urgency, depending upon our current state of health; someone seriously ill from cancer or arthritis is much more vulnerable to toxic overload than, say an Olympic decathlon athlete. Interestingly, however, it could be said that the average Olympic athlete is much more aware and careful about his/her health and environment than the rest of the population. That could be the most eloquent testimony of all to taking responsibility for every aspect of our lifestyle.

Vitamin C: The Master Nutrient

The generous provision of natural antioxidants including vitamin C in one's daily dietary regimen can promote better defense against those all-pervasive destructive free-radical elements emanating from within and without our bodies.

Chapter 6

FIGHTER OF HEART DISEASE AND DIABETES

Heart disease, including heart attack, is the number-one killer in the western world, accounting for 48 percent of all deaths in the U.S. Related conditions to heart disease, including stroke, account for an additional 10 percent of deaths. That means heart disease in one form or another contributes to almost 60 percent of all deaths[166]. And diabetics are more prone than non-diabetics to develop cardiovascular complications, which, as will be discussed later, may have a vitamin C connection[123,167,223].

What contributes most to heart disease are clogged arteries or arteriosclerosis. And what causes clogged, plaque-filled arteries are high lipid and cholesterol levels. What causes high cholesterol levels is eating too much saturated fat. The way to reduce cholesterol levels is to reduce dietary intake of animal fats and dairy products, sources of saturated fat. And so the fable of the last 30 years or so goes on. Right? Not necessarily!

Are you aware that a long-term, large-scale epidemiological study of the population of Framingham, Massachusetts, conducted by the National Institute of Health showed no significant correlation between dietary cholesterol intake and blood cholesterol levels, and that at least eight clinical trials conducted in the U.S., U.K. and Scandinavia between 1965 and 1972 also showed that changing the amount of dietary cholesterol had no significant effect upon heart disease?[3,45,166,240]

Eminent and erudite nutritional physicians such as Dr. George V. Mann of Vanderbilt University School of Medicine have added their voices, through such distinguished journals as the *New England Journal of Medicine*: "Foundations, scientists and the media . . . have promoted low cholesterol, polyunsaturated diets, and yet the epidemic continues unabated . . . the oil and spread industry advertises its products . . . promises that make these foods seem like drugs"[166].

Are you aware that in fact, according to published evidence by Professor John Yudkin, even as long ago as 1957, more than 30 years ago, there is a direct and highly significant correlation between the intake of sugar and heart disease in 15 countries? Clinical and epidemiological studies conducted by Yudkin confirmed that men eating high quantities of sugar were at significantly greater risk of developing heart disease than those with low sugar intakes [243-4]. When has this been publicized in the media?

Several anomalies in the high fat-heart disease story also indicate that sugar, not fat is the main culprit[80], at least among peoples such as Yemenite Jews[57], East

African Masai and Sumburu tribes, all of whom ate a high-fat, low sugar diet and who didn't suffer from heart disease until sugar intake increased[166].

And are you aware that way back in the 1930s, that's 50 years ago, a link between vitamin C and atherosclerosis and heart disease had already been established?[151,174,205] Are you also aware that by 1953, 35 years ago, an intimate relationship between vitamin C, cholesterol synthesis and atherosclerosis had already been documented[18,163,235] and that by 1959, it had been shown that atherosclerosis is reversible by vitamins?[149,236-39] Even as early as 1947 it was suggested in a clinical article[211] that vitamin C be used for treatment of heart disease. Furthermore, vitamin C also possesses significant therapeutic impact upon diabetes and hypoglycemia. But is vitamin C being widely dispensed by cardiovascular specialists and hospitals?[76]

Read today's newspapers. Page 1, Sept. 3, 1989, of the *London Sunday Times*: "Poly Fats Bad for You." *New Scientist,* Sept. 9, 1989: "Media saturation fuels debate about fats in the diet." Full-page ad in *London Observer,* Sept. 10, 1989: "Polyunsaturates are Essential for Health," sponsored by the "Flora Project" (Flora is a brand of margarine).

What's going on here? Is it any wonder that everyone, including the public, is thoroughly confused about what is or isn't good for you? And while we're all bending over backwards to attempt to reduce cholesterol levels by not eating animal and dairy derived fats, is it really to no avail to our improved health? What are the facts, and how can we, as discriminating health-conscious individuals, cut through this massive gobbledygook of scientific and medical red tape? And, furthermore, who can we believe, with so many "experts" lining up on different sides of the heart disease question?

Having surveyed the historical literature concerning heart disease, cholesterol and vitamin C, the author is appalled at this scandalous outrage of reinforced ignorance and misinformation. Fifty years ago is a long time; even 30 years is long ago. But even today in 1990, the public is still being barraged by the media about fat and high cholesterol levels. Something has got to change. And that seems to point to a more highly critical and discerning consumer who is willing to question and doubt even their doctors. In actuality, sober reading of the clinical information about cholesterol, heart disease, and the impact of vitamin C, is lucid, highly revealing, and offers food for thought and helpful suggestions for sufferers of heart-related conditions.

The Cholesterol Story

Consider cholesterol, the lipid substance, formula $C_{27}H_{46}O$. It's found in all bodily tissues, particularly in the brain, spinal cord, liver and bile. The liver manufactures cholesterol, quite a lot of it, about 3/4 g per day, from a variety of sources, including acetate, an organic salt generated during normal metabolism, dietary cholesterol, and bile acids reabsorbed from the intestine[166]. There is actually a cholesterol cycle:

1. Cholesterol is synthesized in the liver;

2. Cholesterol, associated with a lipoprotein called low-density lipoprotein (LDL), is transported through the body's bloodstream. This is the stage of the cycle where cholesterol can attach to and be deposited in the linings of arteries.

3. Cholesterol, associated with another lipoprotein called high-density lipoprotein (HDL), is transported to the gall bladder where it is converted to bile acids, which are then eliminated via the intestines.

4. Some of the bile acids are reabsorbed from the intestines, reconverted to cholesterol and hence carry on with the cholesterol cycle.

The cholesterol that we consume in our diet obviously does constitute part of the cholesterol "pool" in the body; the recommended dietary levels of 25-300 mg would therefore constitute less than 10 percent of the total cholesterol amount made by the liver. Moreover, there is a feedback mechanism which will decrease the amount of newly synthesized cholesterol if we consume more cholesterol than normal[166]. In the above-mentioned Framingham study, there was no difference in the total serum cholesterol levels of the men and women who consumed higher or lower amounts of cholesterol in their diet[166]. Actually, the total amount of cholesterol in the blood is determined by the interaction of four factors:

1. The rate of cholesterol liver synthesis from acetate.

2. The rate of cholesterol obtained from food.

3. The rate of cholesterol converted to bile acids and excreted via the intestines.

4. The rate of bile acids reabsorbed and reconverted to cholesterol.

What becomes crucial in the cholesterol story is the biochemistry and processing of cholesterol in our bodies. High serum cholesterol levels are dangerous, and are correlated with increased risk of heart disease. In a study conducted by the National Heart Institute in which blood cholesterol levels were reduced by 8.5 percent, the death rate from heart disease was reduced by 25 percent[166]. However, dietary sources of cholesterol are not necessarily the principal contributors of total cholesterol levels, and altering dietary cholesterol intake alone does not necessarily produce lower cholesterol levels.

The biochemistry and function of the two lipoproteins, LDL and HDL are crucial in understanding the cholesterol cycle. LDLs, low-density lipoproteins, carry cholesterol throughout the bloodstream, enabling cholesterol to "stick" to cell linings. LDLs are "bad guys". HDLs, on the other hand, transport cholesterol back to the gall bladder, where it is converted to bile acid and excreted via the intestines. HDLs are therefore "good guys," because they are helping to eliminate cholesterol. A growing body of evidence now indicates that total cholesterol, LDL and HDL measurements are actually a more reliable index of our cholesterol "status" than simply total cholesterol measurements alone. High levels of cholesterol and LDL correlate with high risk of heart disease; high levels of HDL correlate with low risk of heart disease.

This is not to deny that the amount and type of fat consumed, whether saturated or polyunsaturated, is not an important parameter in the heart disease equation. The essentiality and benefit to health of certain types of polyunsaturated fats have received considerable attention in recent years as has the potentially increased rate of free radical formation with the use of polyunsaturated fats found in margarine. For a more detailed coverage of the fats and oils story, which is beyond the scope of this volume, the reader is enthusiastically referred to *Fats and Oils* by

Udo Erasmus[74]. For the sugar connection, Yudkin's *Sweet and Dangerous*[244] is highly recommended.

Thus far, the majority of health investigators have concentrated upon the dietary cholesterol factor in the heart disease equation[206]. However, research into other aspects, such as increasing HDL levels and thus the elimination of cholesterol, increasing the synthesis of collagen, a major structural component of blood, and inhibiting the degradation of the lining of arteries, has yielded valuable information which has documented and corroborated the 1930s research which implicated vitamin C deficiencies with heart valve and muscle lesions, and heart disease. In fact, there is now a considerable volume of clinical, biochemical and epidemiological evidence which attests to vitamin C's important role in preventing, controlling and even reversing the number-one killer—heart disease[5,15,18,29,31-2,58,69,76-8,81,131,189,190,195,209,216,223,230]

The Vitamin C–Heart Disease Connection

Clinical and epidemiological studies demonstrate that vitamin C plays a vital role in the prevention, control and even reversibility of atherosclerosis, the "deposition of hard yellow plaques of lipoid material in the intimal layer of the arteries, resulting in arterial degeneration and thickening."

Historically, during the 1930s and 1940s, researchers noted that vitamin deficiencies in guinea pigs led to heart valve and muscle lesions, myocardial degeneration, arteriosclerosis, inflamed heart valves, myocarditis, pericarditis and coronary thrombosis[151,163,174,205,211]; in other words, vitamin C was linked to atherosclerosis. During the 1950s, vitamin C was shown to be related to cholesterol metabolism—

vitamin C deficiency led to increased cholesterol synthesis, feeding animals an increased cholesterol diet reduced vitamin C levels and vitamin C supplementation decreased cholesterol levels[149,235-38]. In 1957, it was discovered (with guinea pigs) that vitamin C could even reverse atherosclerosis[239].

Now, more than 30 years later, our understanding at the biochemical level of how vitamin C protects against heart disease has advanced, along with a concomitant array of epidemiological evidence. Vitamin C has been shown to modulate cholesterol metabolism in the following ways[83-8,157-9,193-6,215]:

1. Vitamin C increases the rate at which cholesterol is removed by its conversion to bile acids and excretion via the intestines;

2. Vitamin C increases HDL levels. High HDL levels are correlated with low risk of heart disease;

3. Vitamin C, through its laxative effect, accelerates elimination of waste, thereby acting to decrease the re-absorption of bile acids and thence their reconversion to cholesterol.

Clinical studies have shown that vitamin C reduces serum cholesterol and triglyceride levels in individuals with high levels. Vitamin C does not reduce cholesterol or triglycerides levels in individuals who are within "normal" values[118], suggesting that vitamin C acts in a homeostatic way to promote equilibrium. For more details on these studies, see the Appendix.

It has been known for over fifty years that vitamin C is essential for the synthesis of collagen[166]. Collagen, a superhelical protein, composed of the amino acids glycine and hydroxyproline, is one of the most important buttresses of the body's structural integrity. Collagen is fibrous and strong, forming the connective tissue essential to strong bones, teeth, skin, muscle, blood vessels—indeed, all body parts[177]. Extensive biochemical research has revealed that vitamin C is required for almost every step involved in the complex synthesis of collagen. Deficiencies of vitamin C lead to a weakening of the structural foundation of all body parts, including blood vessels, the heart and heart muscle[14]. The intimate involvement of vitamin C with collagen synthesis is certainly a factor in C's positive effect in protecting against heart disease[201, 203].

At the molecular level, Dr. Anthony Verlangieri, director of the Atherosclerosis Research Laboratories at the University of Mississippi, and his co-workers have for twenty years been researching the mechanisms behind vitamin C's therapeutic effect upon atherosclerosis[219]. Dr. Verlangieri has shown that vitamins C and E are required for the synthesis of a substance called glycosaminoglycan (GAG), a crucial ingredient of the "cement" that holds arterial cells in place[224]. Deficiencies of vitamin C lead to deterioration of the cell lining, resulting in arterial lesions, which can then fill up with cholesterol, causing atherosclerosis[223]. The mechanisms of vitamin C's role in GAG synthesis have been elucidated by Verlangieri's group.

Additional studies have also demonstrated that arteries with high vitamin C levels have lower cholesterol levels and that vitamins C and E can actually reverse the disease process of atherosclerosis[230]! See Fig. 4 in the Appendix.

Vitamin C: The Master Nutrient

Vitamin C Prolongs Life: Epidemiological Evidence

Epidemiological studies provide the final proof of which factors are statistically correlated with the hypothesis in question. Several epidemiological studies performed with vitamin C in America, the UK and throughout Europe provide evidence that vitamin C has an important protective effect against heart disease. In fact, one study by Chope and Breslow[55] reveals that vitamin C supplementation was the most important factor in decreasing the death rate.

A study by Gey et al.[82] recently presented at the Third Conference on Vitamin C surveyed the plasma levels of vitamin C of populations at different risks from heart disease throughout Europe, including southern Italy, Switzerland, Northern Ireland, Scotland and two regions in Finland. The results, shown in Fig. 5 in the Appendix, were highly revealing and demonstrated the important protective factor that vitamin C represents against ischemic heart disease (IHD).

In southern Italy and Switzerland, where vitamin C levels were adequate, the heart disease mortality was low. In Northern Ireland, where vitamin C levels were on the borderline between adequate and marginally deficient, the heart disease mortality was medium. In Scotland, where heart disease mortality was high, vitamin C levels actually dipped into the region of being at risk for overt scurvy. This study also showed the protective effect of vitamin E against heart disease.

Vitamin C to Replace Triple Bypass Surgery?

The research data has certainly been accumulating in favor of vitamin C's powerful effects in reducing cholesterol and LDL, increasing HDL levels, actually reversing the atherosclerotic process, and in decreasing mortality from heart disease in a variety of populations from Western countries. Will we be seeing the day when safe, inexpensive vitamin C may replace dangerous and expensive surgical treatment such as open heart surgery to clear arteries clogged by cholesterol? In this instance, surely the saying "An ounce of prevention is worth a pound of cure" is more than apt when it comes to vitamin C and heart disease.

The Diabetes Connection

Diabetics are at greater risk of suffering the complications of heart disease and atherosclerosis. Despite the life-saving effects of insulin in preventing diabetic coma, diabetics suffer secondary complications such as blindness and atherosclerosis. These complications include a 25-fold greater incidence of retinal artery disease, a seven-fold greater incidence of kidney disease and a high incidence of coronary arterial conditions[221,223].

One explanation of this high incidence of cardiovascular disease among diabetics invokes the molecular similarity of glucose and vitamin C, discussed in Chapter 3. In diabetes, there is an insufficient level of the hormone insulin to uptake glucose from the blood into cells. Therefore, although the diabetic may have extremely high glucose levels in the blood and urine, his cells may actually be starved for glucose, because they need insulin to transport glucose into the cell.

Since vitamin C is structurally very similar to glucose, one of the transport mechanisms of vitamin C into the cells has been suggested to be via the insulin transport mechanism. If, as in diabetes, glucose concentrations are very high, then vitamin C will be "out-competed" by glucose and will simply not get into the cells. As stated by Pecoraro and Chen[167], who were investigating competition for membrane transport between glucose and ascorbic acid, at the most recent Vitamin C International Conference, "These results are consistent with the hypothesis that chronic hyperglycemia may be associated with intracellular deficits of leukocyte ascorbic acid, an impaired acute inflammatory response, and altered susceptibility to infection and faulty wound repair in patients with diabetes."

This cellular deficiency in vitamin C, with its concomitant effects—increased cholesterol levels, increased atherosclerosis degeneration of heart and arterial tissues—contribute to the above-named complications experienced by diabetics[191].

Vitamin C is said to be a potentizer of insulin, in that less insulin is needed to control blood sugar when vitamin C is given in combination[180,198]. If it's true that the complications of diabetes are the result of cellular vitamin C deficiency, then treatment aimed at increasing vitamin C levels in diabetics ought to yield beneficial therapeutic effects.

There has already accumulated a considerable clinical literature linking vitamin C with insulin action[11-13,95,169,171,200]. Continued research into the interactions of vitamin C and insulin may yield a safe and inexpensive way to control diabetes and to prevent the development of the tragic cardiovascular complications suffered by millions of diabetics.

Chapter 7

VITAMIN C AND ARTHRITIS

Arthritis is the archetype of a holistic disease. It is not a single, simple condition; in fact, although rheumatoid arthritis and osteoarthritis constitute the two largest classes of joint diseases, the family of more than 100 types of arthritis may be associated with other systemic diseases and deficiencies, as shown in Table 7 in the Appendix.

Arthritis is not caused or treated by a single agent. Complex interrelated contributory factors to this most painful and dreaded disease may include:

Infectious microorganisms such as viruses, bacteria and protozoa;
Physical injuries to bones and joints;
Nutritional deficiencies of protein, minerals and vitamins;
Toxic environmental pollutants;

Metabolic and immunological disorders, including
   allergies;
Psychological and emotional stress.

   Tens of millions of people suffer the outrageous
slings and arrows of arthritis, desperate for and
bereft of any hope of relief or cure. Victims of seemingly unbearable pain, arthritic sufferers have classi-
cally been condemned to the medical merry-go-
round of the toxic arthritic drug emporium: aspirin,
cortisone, non-steroidal anti-inflammatory agents
(NSAIDS), gold shots, penicillamine, methotrexate
and, as a last resort, surgery.

The side effects of all these traditional anti-arthritic
drugs can be severe:

   Aspirin: gastric bleeding, stomach upset, loss of
      hearing, tinnitus, increased bleeding time, aller-
      gic reactions
   Corticosteroids: suppression of immune response,
      "moon-face," bruising, psychic derangements, cat-
      aracts, glaucoma, ocular infection, elevated blood
      pressure, salt and water retention
   NSAIDS: gastric, nervous, hepatic, skin, renal, oc-
      ular and blood disorders
   Gold: bone marrow damage, anemia, exfoliative
      dermatitis
   Penicillamine: generalized allergic reactions, gas-
      trointestinal pain, nausea, vomiting, diarrhea,
      peptic ulcer, liver dysfunction, pancreatitis, bone
      marrow depression, aplastic anemia, renal dys-
      function and/or failure, tinnitus, myasthenia gra-
      vis. Penicillamine is a drug with a high incidence

of severe reactions, some of which are potentially fatal.

Methotrexate: bone marrow damage, anemia, leukopenia, bleeding, extensive liver damage, fetal deaths, congenital anomalies, diarrhea, ulcerative stomatitis, hemorrhagic enteritis and death from intestinal perforation

Fortunately, there is good news, thanks in very large measure to the painstaking and pioneering work worldwide, of over 200 physicians in 15 different countries who have each contributed innovative and effective treatments in the development and implementation of an integrated and comprehensive program to fight and win the battle with arthritis.

Physicians who pioneered and developed the Rheumatoid Disease Foundation's recommendations, which have since 1982 produced a consistent 80 percent remission/cure rate for so-called intransigent rheumatoid diseases, include Drs. Roger Wyburn-Mason and Paul Pybus, both now deceased, Jack M. Blount, Gus J. Prosch, along with outstanding contributions by many others. Central to these successes has been: (1) the use of certain oral medications; (2) intraneural injections; (3) appropriate diet and supplements; and (4) other appropriate treatments, such as treatment for Candidiasis, virtually universal in arthritics.

The Rheumatoid Disease Foundation has published several outstandingly written volumes describing this comprehensive arthritis regime for the layman, which combines all modalities of treatment: physical, nutritional, infectious, emotional and spiritual. Several, which are highly recommended reading for everyone, include: *The Art of Getting Well,* Anthony Di Fabio, 1988[71]; *Fight Back Against Arthritis,* Robert Bingham, 1985[21]; and *Rheumatoid Diseases— Cured At Last,* Anthony Di Fabio, 1982[70]. These books provide a wealth of well-presented information relating to cause, diagnosis, treatment, diet, counselling, and exercises for the entire range of arthritic conditions.

Why Vitamin C?

Vitamin C is vital to any arthritic therapeutic program, because vitamin C has an intimate therapeutic relationship with each of the major causes of arthritis: physical structure of joints and bones (collagen); immune response against infectious agents; nutritional deficiency; and stress.

As can be recalled from previous chapters, vitamin C is a requirement for almost every step in the synthesis of collagen, that fibrous protein which forms the strong connective tissue vital for strong bones, cartilage, the very bodily structures which become degenerate in arthritic diseases. Hence, vitamin C must figure prominently in any health-promoting and arthritis-prevention program in order for wound healing and regeneration of connective tissues to proceed at optimal levels.

As related in the preceding chapter, arteriosclerosis (the clogging of arteries with cholesterol) interferes with normal circulation and metabolism of bones and joints, leading to degeneration and ultimately to arthritis. The previously described sterling role of vitamin C in the prevention and even reversal of arteriosclerosis is yet another strong indication of the role of vitamin C in the prevention and treatment of arthritis.

The role of vitamin C in maintaining and strengthening immune resistance to infectious agents, and especially in the function of particular white cells, is yet another facet of vitamin C's power against arthritis. Considerable research points to a pivotal role played by microorganisms in arthritis. Vitamin C's multi-faceted role in stimulating lymphocyte production, modulating the levels of circulating antibodies, in the synthesis of complement, the production of the body's natural anti-viral substance interferon, in the inhibition of the prostaglandins involved in inflammatory responses—swelling, pain, tenderness and heat—and vitamin C's salutary therapeutic effects in allergic responses (often a critical component of arthritis) all speak to vitamin C's essential role in the successful treatment of arthritis.

Ester-C Ascorbate's Therapeutic Success in Arthritis

The majority of physicians working with arthritic sufferers develop treatment regimes to alleviate the pain in the individual. It's difficult to set up controlled cross-over trials to assess the effectiveness of various treatments and, as a result, most available information is anecdotal and subjective. Countless case histories exist detailing the effects of Ester-C ascorbate; the following represents a small sample exerpted from one doctor's files.

Dr. Edwin Goertz, a Canadian-trained physician with a distinguished medical career in Canada and the United States in Emergency Medicine, Rehabilitation Medicine and private practice, has used Ester-C with 300 arthritic patients. Dr. Goertz reports[90]:

... at least 50 percent have consistently reported beneficial results in their symptoms using Ester-C either as a primary treatment or as adjunctive therapy. Also I have never observed any toxic side effects to this product or had any adverse reactions when taken in conjunction with other medications

Several case histories are hereby appended:

Female, age 61. Diagnosis, osteoarthritis of many years affecting major joints and back. Patient had very limited success with various arthritis medications and treatment. She was placed on Ester-C ascorbate t.i.d. (three times per day) along with calcium salicylate 800 mg t.i.d. She was virtually free of pain for one and a half months until she incurred back strain. For a brief time she ran out of Ester-C ascorbate and substituted vitamin C with immediate exacerbation of pain. Patient insisted on remaining on Ester-C during the past year and has experienced no side effects.

Female, age 83. Diagnosis of degenerative joint disease most severe in hips and knees. Had history of intolerance to most arthritic medication and little or no relief from salicylates. Was placed on Ester-C ascorbate t.i.d. and calcium salicylate 800 mg. t.i.d. for two weeks. She reported improved knee pain especially during the night.

Female, age 66. Diagnosis of rheumatoid arthritis with extensive deformities as a child. Patient was placed on Ester-C 300 mg. t.i.d. She felt much improved in a few days both physically and mentally and was able to reduce Prednisone and analgesics to about one-half dosage. She commented,

Vitamin C: The Master Nutrient

"I didn't believe I could ever feel this good again." Patient has remained on Ester-C during the past year with continued benefit and no side effects.

Male, age 60. Diagnosis of osteoarthritis with symptoms primarily of hands. Ester-C three times a day with moderate improvement in pain over three-week period. The patient then discontinued Ester-C and noticed an increase in pain. He then resumed Ester-C with a notable improvement.

Male, age 55. Degenerative arthritis in the knees for several years with occasional edema at times but fairly persistent pain. At time of initial consult there was mild joint effusion and tenderness of left knee. Placed on Ester-C three times daily. On three months follow–up almost asymptomatic with no other medications but Ester-C and working as full-time truck driver.

Crippled Dogs Walk Again

Over the last 30 years, Draconian efforts have been undertaken by breeders and veterinarians to eliminate canine hip dysplasia. These measures included sterilization of all pups from a dysplastic litter and selective breeding of only those dogs free from hip dysplasia. These strategies were ineffective, since they were based on the erroneous assumption that canine hip dysplasia is an inherited birth defect. More recent clinical research[20] demonstrates that canine hip dysplasia develops as a result of inadequate vitamin C in the young puppy, resulting in poor-quality, low-strength collagen in the affected ligaments. Although dogs produce their own vitamin C, certain breeds produce low levels of vitamin C, insufficient to counter the high levels of stress encountered in early life. Vitamin C is essential in the synthesis of collagen, the building blocks of muscles, ligaments, bones and tendons. Over the past five years, eight litters of German shepherd puppies from parents with hip dysplasia have been totally devoid of canine hip dysplasia under the following regime: the pregnant bitch is administered 2 to 4 g vitamin C daily; from birth to 3 weeks, the pups are given 50 to 100 mg vitamin C orally; from 3 weeks until 4 months, 500 mg; from 4 months to 2 years, 1 to 2 gm daily. See the Appendix for more study results.

The possible mechanisms for Ester-C ascorbate appearing to exert a therapeutic effect in arthritis, beyond that of vitamin C^6, are presently not fully understood. However, the case of the dogs' (who, of course, manufacture their own vitamin C) recovery from their chronic ailments[73,156] in response to Ester-C supplementation, is quite dramatic evidence that possibly the metabolites in Ester-C exert a yet-to-be-discovered powerful therapeutic effect. More rigorous clinical trials with these dogs are presently in progress in Norway.

Treatment Programs for Arthritis

The author wishes to point out that vitamin C should be regarded as merely one component of a fully comprehensive program in the treatment of arthritis. The type(s) of arthritis should be established by careful diagnosis. This program, following the guidelines set out by the Rheumatoid Disease Foundation, should consist of anti-protozoal treatments, and individualized nutritional program paying

Vitamin C: The Master Nutrient

careful attention to allergies, nutritional supplements including vitamin C, exercise, relaxation and emotional support. Additional complementary treatments such as hydrotherapy and acupuncture may also be appropriate.

Chapter 8

VITAMIN C AND CANCER

Some two years ago, while visiting my family in Montreal, I had the devastating experience of witnessing my Aunt Kate's painful hospital ordeal with cancer. Subjected to cytotoxic treatments of radiation therapy and dosed with narcotics to control the pain, poor Kate, always such a jovial and cheerful dear soul, appeared to wander in and out of consciousness. She finally died several months later, having been able to return home for a brief few months.

My family is very traditional and has absolute faith in the medical profession. In their opinion, if vitamins and diet could help, they would be prescribed by their doctor. To see someone I loved dearly dying and not be able to mitigate some of the toxic effects of the hospital/medical regime with immune-enhancing natural medicines and nutrients such as vitamin C underscores for me how radically attitudes must

71

change before our health care system freely and openly embraces the best of all traditions.

The so-called "war against cancer" has drained billions of dollars, created illusions of miracle cures in the public eye, while harassing and prosecuting those vanguard physicians courageous enough to discover, research or treat cancer patients with nontraditional medicines. The so-called "progress" of the past few decades includes: the prosecution in the U.S. of pioneering cancer giants such as Drs. Lawrence Burton, Emanuel Revici and Stanislaw Burzynski[110]; the subjection of nearly 50 percent of all cancer patients to toxic chemotherapy which has been shown to objectively help only 5 percent[56]; the denial of research grants to study the action of alternative cancer treatments; the shoddy research which has been carried out by certain institutions to supposedly investigate the therapeutic efficacy of nutrients such as vitamin C[166]. At least one group, Project Cure[172], has formed an effective lobby to promote and advocate research and access to alternative cancer treatments in response.

Here are the facts:

1. Twenty years ago the chance of getting cancer was one in six; now it is one in three.

2. Traditional cancer treatments, i.e. surgery, radiation and chemotherapy, which have improved the management and prognosis of certain cancers, have not measured up to expectations of affording a cure for cancer, and have often worsened the misery of cancer patients through their toxic effects[9,56].

3. Data is accumulating which shows that a high proportion of cancers are at the very least influenced or aggravated by environmental factors: stress, high

sugar, high fat, refined diet, smoking, alcohol, pollu-tion, and carcinogenic substances we ingest through the food we eat or the chemicals we handle in our work[56].

4. It is possible to positively enhance the quality of life and often our survival[154] with cancer, through the judicious use of positive mental attitude[100], a nutritious diet and exercise program, and supple-mentation with high doses of certain health-enhancing and detoxifying nutrients such as vitamin C[40-44,154].

Vitamin C and its effects upon many types of cancer have been studied in animals and in humans over the past 30 years. The preoccupation of the medical research establishment with more high-tech and profitable treatments has not afforded the ex-tensive research into non-toxic substances such as vitamin C which could have been accomplished over this time period.

There is, nevertheless, a respectable body of evi-dence which documents the therapeutic effects of vitamin C on cancer which are briefly summarized here:

1. Vitamin C delays the appearance of breast tumor formation in mice from six weeks to 120 weeks[165].

2. Plasma levels of vitamin C are inversely corre-lated with incidence of gastrointestinal and cervical cancers[23,181,232].

3. Vitamin C detoxifies carcinogenic nitrites and nitrates[54,204].

4. Vitamin C acts synergistically with radiation treatment for cervical cancer[54,181,232].

5. Vitamin C prevents formation of bladder tumors[166].

6. Vitamin C inhibits the action of hyaluronidase (the enzyme found in malignant tumors), thereby slowing down the degradation of cellular tissues and invasion by cancerous growths[43,44].

7. Vitamin C controls pain in cancer patients to such an extent that morphine and other narcotic pain-relieving drugs are often not needed[43,44].

8. Vitamin C increases the sense of well-being, and hence the quality of life of cancer patients[43,44].

9. A decrease in malignant cells shed from tumors is seen[166].

10. There is some reversal from hepatomegaly (enlargement of the liver) and malignant jaundice[166].

11. There is a decline in the red blood cell sedimentation rate[166].

12. Vitamin C counteracts many of the unpleasant side effects of chemotherapy[43].

13. Vitamin C stimulates the production of phagocytic leukocytes, white blood cells active in engulfing and destroying cancerous cells[242].

14. Vitamin C destroys free radicals, which have been seriously implicated in cancer formation[7,161,182].

The Clinical Evidence

Dr. Ewan Cameron, Senior Consultant Surgeon in Vale of Leven Hospital, Scotland, has been treating "hopeless" and "terminal"cancer patients for over 15 years with vitamin C, 10 g or more per day[40-44]. With his growing experience with hundreds of such patients, whose lives have been extended and improved, he has accumulated considerable evidence of vitamin C's efficacy against cancer. Due to his self-professed "bias" that vitamin C definitely prolongs the life of cancer patients, Dr. Cameron has shunned, on ethical grounds, the conducting of double-blind, placebo-controlled trials, because he would not want to deny a single cancer patient the option to take vitamin C just for the advancement of research. However, Dr. Cameron has in fact conducted several trials in which he has compared the treatment of 100 vitamin C cancer patients with 1,000 matched controls—that is, patients of the same age group, cancer type, treatment, diet, everything, that is, except vitamin C.

In one such study by Dr. Cameron, published in 1976, all 1,000 control patients had died, while 18/100 of the vitamin C-treated patients were still alive[41]. In fact, the vitamin C-treated patients lived 300 days longer than the controls! In 1978, a similar study divided the patients into eight groups of different types of cancer: ovary, rectum, bronchus, stomach, colon, bladder, kidney and breast. The vitamin C group lived from 114–435 days longer than the control group. Eight percent of the vitamin C patients were alive, while none of the controls were[42].

The Mayo Clinic "carefully controlled trials" of 1979 and 1985[61,153], which, amidst considerable publicity, refuted any therapeutic claim for vitamin C and cancer, were seriously flawed in several respects:

1. Most of the Mayo patients had received cytotoxic chemotherapy for their cancer prior to vitamin C. Chemotherapy drugs destroy the immune system, thereby making it more difficult for immune-enhancing agents such as vitamin C to act.

2. The "control" group of Mayo patients was taking vitamin C in not insignificant dosages, invalidating this group as a control.

75

3. The vitamin C group only received vitamin C for a short time—two and a half months—after which time the treatment was suspended. Dr. Cameron's patients took vitamin C every day for the rest of their lives.

The Epidemiological Evidence

A Johns Hopkins study conducted by Wassertheil-Smoller[232], with 169 women investigated for cervical dysplasias (abnormalities) indicated that women with low plasma levels of vitamin C stand a ten-fold increased risk of cervical dysplasia. Another American study conducted by Romney et al.[181] found low vitamin C levels in asymptomatic women with cervical carcinoma in situ.

A Norwegian and American study conducted in 1973 and 74 by Bjelke[23], surveying 30,000 people, showed a negative correlation between vitamin C and gastric cancer. A more recent study by Stahelin et al.[197] corroborated this inverse correlation of vitamin C with gastric cancer, and furthermore documented that vitamin C appears to act synergistically with other factors (most notably smoking and alcohol) in its action against cancer. Vitamins A, E and other antioxidants also show an inverse relationship with gastric cancer.

The Role of Vitamin C in Cancer Treatment

Vitamin C is recommended as an adjunct and integral component of any cancer regime, not as the sole treatment for cancer. Vitamin C has been shown to enhance and potentiate the effects of traditional cancer treatments, including radiation and chemotherapy. Since every cancer is unique, an individualized treatment program, incorporating the mind and spirit (stress reduction, positive imaging), and the body (nutrition, supplements, medicines) will have the greatest successful effects in the treatment of cancer.

Chapter 9

ATTACK ON VIRUSES

Vitamin C and Colds

The advocacy of vitamin C for the prevention and treatment of colds has received more publicity than perhaps any other health-related subject. Since the publication of Linus Pauling's book *Vitamin C, the Common Cold and the Flu* (1970, Freeman & Co.)[164], debates on the merits and appropriate doses of vitamin C have raged within the research establishment and among the public. Despite such universal bombardment via every kind of media, old ideas die hard; it continually astonishes me how a majority of people, convinced that the body "only stores 150 mg vitamin C and excretes the rest," content themselves with rather small doses (500 mg a day) and wonder why they haven't experienced the wondrous effects of vitamin C rhapsodized by enthusiastic advocates.

The research history concerning the use of vitamin C against colds and viruses is actually almost half a century old. The detailed historical description of the various research trials conducted since the 1940s makes compelling reading, and the reader is enthusiastically encouraged to review the evidence presented by Drs. Irwin Stone and Linus Pauling in their respective books[164,166,200]. A summary of placebo-controlled trials with vitamin C and colds (Table 5) is hereby reprinted from Dr. Pauling's *How to Live Longer and Feel Better*, 1986[166]:

Table 5.
Controlled Studies Related to Vitamin C and Colds

STUDY	% DECREASE IN ILLNESS PER PERSON
Glacebrook & Thomson (1942)	50
Cowan, Diehl, Baker (1942)	31
Dahlberg, Engel, Rydin (1944)	14
Franz, Sands, Heyl (1954)	36
Anderson et al. (1975)	25
Ritzel (1961)	63
Anderson, Reid, Beaton (1972)	32
Charleston, Clegg (1972)	58
Elliott (1973)	44
Anderson, Suranyi, Beaton (1974)	9
Coulehan et al. (1974)	30
Sabiston & Radomski (1974)	68
Karlowski et al. (1975)	21
Clegg & Macdonald (1975)	8
Pitt & Costrini (1979)	0
Carr et al. (1981)	48
Average Percentage Decrease	35

From *How to Live longer and Feel Better*, Linus Pauling, 1986[166]

Vitamin C: The Master Nutrient

It should be borne in mind that none of the above studies really tested vitamin C's effect against colds to the limit, in that the above studies used relatively low doses for relatively short time intervals. The types of data that would be really convincing would use doses of 3 to 5 g per day over an extended period of time, at least one year.

The Vitamin C Recipe Against Colds

Depending on your biochemical individuality, your own protective dose of vitamin C which should prevent colds may range from 1 to 3 to 5 g per day. However, as will be discussed, this level will vary according to the degree of stresses in your life, including physical, infectious, environmental and emotional. Generally, a "maintenance" dose of vitamin C should offer significant protection against colds. However, when your resistance is lowered due to any number of factors, this is what to do with respect to vitamin C. This regime is again borrowed from Drs. Stone and Pauling[164,166,200]:

1. At the first signs of cold, i.e. scratchy or sore throat, malaise, sniffles, fever, etc., take 1 to 2 g vitamin C. It's important to "catch" the cold at the onset, not to wait until it takes hold.

2. Repeat taking 1 to 2 g vitamin C about every hour. Usually, after several hours, symptoms subside and relief is felt. Take a total of 5 to 20 g vitamin C per day, depending on the severity of symptoms. A very severe cold may require more vitamin C, perhaps as much as 50 to 100 g. To be more precise, what you are trying to achieve is to take vitamin C to "bowel tolerance level," the

optimum level for vitamin C's efficacy. More about this later.

3. Continue taking 5 to 20 g vitamin C for an extended period beyond that of the cold. Symptoms may return if the vitamin C is suddenly withdrawn or reduced too early. Taper off the dosage gradually, until at your maintenance dose of 1 to 3 to 5 g per day. For instance, if you were taking 2 g vitamin C seven times per day, for a total of 14 g per day, after a week, take 2 five times per day for two days, then 2 g four times per day, then 2 g three times per day, then perhaps down to your regular regime of 1.5 g three times per day.

For the die-hard skeptic who never believes any of the experts, this is your opportunity to test the vitamin C cold-fighting recipe for yourself. One of the best attributes about vitamin C is that no matter how much you take, even 200 g per day, it cannot harm you. The clinical evidence of tens of thousands of patients attests to the nontoxicity of vitamin C. There is many a vitamin C supporting individual who started off attempting to disprove the theory that vitamin C can prevent and treat colds and other illnesses.

Vitamin C and Other Viral Diseases

Historically (virtually as soon as viruses were first identified) published research reports vitamin C's potent broad-spectrum anti-viral activity against a wide range of different viruses. Table 8 in the Appendix highlights this very early research, going back over 50 years ago.

Although research decades ago documented the potent force of vitamin C as a viral inhibitor, this has

Vitamin C: The Master Nutrient

not been taken up by mainstream clinical or pharmacological concerns, who have spent billions in attempting to produce vaccines. And in 1989 vitamin C was shown to inhibit HIV virus, the virus implicated in AIDS.

Chapter 10

VITAMIN C AND METABOLITES KILL THE AIDS VIRUS

Acquired Immunodeficiency Syndrome (AIDS) has become the ultimate horror story, affecting the entire world. Before AIDS, cancer was *the* dread, often unmentionable, disease—it still is, but AIDS is having a uniquely horrible impact. AIDS, in a period of less than one decade, has not only claimed the lives of thousands around the world, but has managed to alter radically social practices and attitudes on sex and relationships. It has virtually reinstated non-promiscuity and fidelity, as well as promoting the widespread use of condoms to such an extent that they are available in vending machines in women's as well as men's washrooms. Such is the terror of AIDS that more than 32 countries now require long-term visitors to produce recent evidence of not being infected with HIV, the human immunodeficiency virus.

Vitamin C: The Master Nutrient

AIDS is the result of an immune system devastated by HIV and presumably other co-factors, which leave the individual vulnerable to potentially fatal attack even by normally innocuous agents. And as the person's immune system gradually weakens, so does his or her resistance to disease. AIDS is insidious, since the very cells designed to protect you from disease are those targeted for destruction by HIV.

Everything about AIDS is controversial—its hypothesized origins, the causative organism or organisms, the drugs and treatments being developed, the methods of testing these treatments, the widespread consumer-driven impulse to use alternative AIDS treatments, the social attitudes toward HIV-infected persons, even institutional attitudes of giant insurance companies toward AIDS patients[147]. And the wastage and horror of AIDS is being indelibly inscribed on our consciousness as increasing numbers of friends, relatives and acquaintances are touched by this latter-day plague.

The battles rage among the scientific and medical experts about every aspect of AIDS, even whether HIV is the cause of the disease or merely a co-factor. The medical establishment sees infection with HIV as leading inevitably to death, whereas "alternative" practitioners (including many MDs) report cases of individuals who have seemingly beaten the virus and are healthy even 8 to 10 years after infection. Even amidst suffering and death, sagas of tremendous spiritual insight and growth with AIDS victims and their caregivers abound. And despite the billions of dollars being expended on AIDS research, the eventual control of this worldwide epidemic will, in this author's opinion, be more the combined result of sensible lifestyle changes and natural evolutionary alterations in the virulence of HIV than any impressive technological marvels— not to say that an effective vaccine would not also be invaluable!

As usual, vitamin C is right in the thick of these battles. Considerable persistence and effort was required before the research descried in this chapter documenting vitamin C's inhibition of HIV was accepted for publication by a scholarly scientific journal. The field of AIDS research is a highly charged political arena, with scientific reputations, budgets and potential Nobel Prizes at stake. Billions are being spent in the academic and corporate sectors on the development of drugs and vaccines against AIDS.

Several years ago, physicians Robert Cathcart[47-48] of the U.S. and Ian Brighthope[35] of Australia reported the clinically effective use of vitamin C in treating AIDS patients, who were staying alive twice as long and suffering many less infections and symptoms of AIDS. The report that a natural, inexpensive and unpatentable substance such as vitamin C could be highly potent and effective against AIDS may represent a threat as well as an embarrassment to the drug companies, which may suffer considerable financial losses with failure and/or toxicity of their own drugs.

The research reported here for the first time outside of the scientific journals, performed at the Linus Pauling Institute, had the blessing and cooperation of one of the scientific pioneers of AIDS research, Dr. Robert Gallo, who supplied the first batches of chronically infected cell lines used. In addition, the research received the enthusiastic support of Dr. Michael McGrath of San Francisco General Hospital, who provided another batch of the same cell line. Identical results were obtained by the Pauling Institute investigators with both batches of cells. The molecular biology experiments described here elegantly and rigorously show that vitamin C in the test tube inhibits HIV reverse transcriptase (RT) activity by over 99 percent[97]. Clinical experience with hundreds of AIDS patients with vitamin C also strongly suggests its potential therapeutic effect on this disease. What follows from here on is in the hands of clinicians, politicians and patients

Vitamin C/AIDS Research from the Linus Pauling Institute

The following research was conducted by Drs. S. Harakeh and R. J. Jariwalla and published in 1990[97]. Principal investigator Dr. Jariwalla, currently Director of the Viral Carcinogenesis and Immunodeficiency Program at the Linus Pauling Institute, received his doctorate in virology at the Medical College of Wisconsin and did postdoctoral training in basic cancer research at Johns Hopkins University. Dr. Jariwalla and colleagues are credited with the discovery of cancer-inducing elements from herpes and other viruses. Dr. Jariwalla directs projects related to mechanisms of cancer induction as well as nutritionally related investigations, including the potential role of vitamin C in AIDS[117] and plant-derived phytate in cancer and atherogenesis.

Vitamin C Significantly Inhibits HIV Reverse Transcriptase Activity.

The AIDS virus is called a *retrovirus* because its genetic material is composed of RNA which gets copied into DNA in order for it to function and replicate within the host cell. To accomplish this, HIV is equipped with an enzyme called, logically enough, *reverse transcriptase* (RT). One of the parameters molecular biologists use to assess HIV replication or infectivity is the measurement of HIV RT activity. In one of the experiments reported, a chronically HIV-infected cell line was cultured either with or without the addition of varying levels of vitamin C (0-150 μg/ml), and the level of RT activity determined at differing time periods (0-4 days). In control cells not treated with vitamin C, the level of RT activity started to rise on day 2, reaching a peak on day 4. In sharp contrast, infected cells treated with vitamin C showed markedly inhibited RT activity. By day 2, RT activity was inhibited by more than 90% at vitamin C concentrations greater than 100 μ/ml; by day 4, at 150 μg/ml vitamin C, RT activity was inhibited by greater than 99%[97]! (Fig. 6, Appendix.) Control experiments had previously determined that cell viability was normal at these vitamin C concentrations, i.e., that vitamin C itself was not toxic to these cells. In addition it was shown that at concentrations at which ascorbate inhibited HIV RT, no adverse effects were seen on host metabolic activity and rate of protein synthesis[97].

Vitamin C Inhibits Expression of HIV p24 Antigen.

When the HIV virus infects a cell, it "highjacks" the cell's protein-manufacturing apparatus to start churning out its (HIV's) own proteins. Another indication, in addition to RT activity described above, used by scientists to assess HIV infection, is the expression of p24 antigen, one of the virus's core proteins. Again, as with the previously described experiment, control cells not treated with vitamin C showed an increase in p24 levels on day 2, reaching a peak on day 4. And again, in sharp contrast to control cell culture and those treated with vitamin C, p24 levels were inhibited by almost 90%[97] (Fig. 7, Appendix.) Since control experiments conducted determined that cellular metabolic activity and protein synthesis were not affected in the presence of vitamin C[97], the observed suppression of RT and p24 must be due to inhibition of a specific step or steps in HIV replication. These results are summarized in Table 9 in the Appendix.

Mechanisms of Vitamin C's Inhibition of HIV

Does vitamin C act directly upon HIV, or is there some indirect process of inactivation? Experiments conducted to address this question determined that vitamin C does not directly inactivate the virus nor prevent infection of cells; however, the inhibition of HIV by vitamin C was due to vitamin C's action upon the virus, not upon other cellular processes.

The actual mechanism responsible for vitamin C's anti-HIV properties is not currently known. Further research is continuing to unravel the molecular action of ascorbate on HIV.

Preliminary Clinical Evidence of Vitamin C's Efficacy Against AIDS

Dr. Robert Cathcart has treated hundreds of AIDS patients using large doses (oral and intravenous) of vitamin C. In Dr. Cathcart's words, "Ascorbate, by making short work of colds and other minor infections, and by reducing the duration and complications of major infections, reduces the activation of T-helper cells and thereby slows the multiplication of viruses"[48]. Dr. Ian Brighthope, also successfully using vitamin C to treat AIDS, finds that it ameliorates depressed mental states as well as the bacterial and viral infections associated with AIDS[35]. The results of Drs. Harake and Jariwalla[97], demonstrating HIV suppression by ascorbate in vitro, provide support for a third possibility, that vitamin C may directly block HIV replication in infected cells.

Attempts to conduct controlled clinical trials of vitamin C have been frustrated by the refusal of granting agencies to fund such necessary research. Dr. Brighthope writes that his application to the Research Grants Division of the Commonwealth Department of Health was refused "on the grounds that there was no evidence that vitamin C had any effect on the course of the disease." Attitudes of the National Institutes of Health (NIH) and the MRC in the UK convey similar conservative and intransigent views. The positive therapeutic effect (albeit anecdotal) of nontoxic vitamin C in the treatment of AIDS certainly represents a major step forward and offers advantages over currently available AZT, which is highly toxic and only inhibits new HIV infection.

The inability to obtain funding to conduct clinical trials for natural medicines in treating AIDS is widespread, and has been reported by many researchers, including this author, working with a variety of substances. To the author's knowledge, the only clinical

Vitamin C: The Master Nutrient

trial being conducted today with vitamin C on AIDS is a privately funded effort coordinated by Dr. Russell Jaffe, formerly a senior researcher and clinician at the NIH, now director of Serammune Physicians Lab in Vienna, Virginia.

Chapter 11

THE NEW SUPER C

Many of us harbor stereotyped notions about the process of scientific discovery, images fostered and reinforced by the chronically theatrical and melodramatic media. We conjure up extreme visions ranging from the diabolical, mad scientist, so obsessed with research that no time is left even for eating or other "normal" activities, to the opposite boring image of the spectacled, white-coated automaton, incapable of uttering phrases other than complex equations and Einsteinian theories, devoid of all feeling.

These far-fetched beliefs about scientists and their work would be quickly replaced by a more authentic picture by spending time in any university laboratory concerned with biology, chemistry or physics, and observing the characteristics and quirks of the researchers working on their respective problems.

Vitamin C: The Master Nutrient

Scientific research and discovery are about solving problems and puzzles. When the problem has been solved, the results of any discoveries then become part of a manufacturing or production process, which ought to be methodical and reproducible. However, like writing a book, designing a building, painting or sculpting, scientific discovery is often helped along by other, non-logical factors such as luck, serendipity, talent, hard work, frustration, failure and persistence, the all-too-familiar societal attributes that shape the landscape of human endeavor.

Those who have studied chemistry may have heard the story of Kekulé, who, falling asleep in front of the fire, dreamed about tails of fire chasing each other in a circle; thus was conceived the theory of resonance for structures such as the benzene ring. We have already seen in an earlier chapter how Szent-Györgyi isolated vitamin C without originally intending to do so. In a logical world, one might think that companies would set out to develop a better product than those available in the market. However, more often the most highly original products develop from extremely unlikely sources—ideas conceived while waiting at a bus stop, scribbles on restaurant napkins, or simply looking for one thing and inadvertently finding another. The incredibly wasteful amounts of time, money and effort which have been expended on vitamin C research using tiny antiscorbutic doses have produced fairly uninspiring therapeutic results. On the other hand, the dramatic therapeutic successes of vitamin C to date, including the discovery of the metabolites of Ester-C ascorbate, have been due to inspiration, creativity, hard work and serendipity.

The story of Ester-C ascorbate started with a small company now called Inter-Cal Corporation in Prescott, Arizona, which utilized a new process in the manufacture of calcium ascorbate. This process, in contrast to other methods of ascorbate production[184], does not use solvents such as alcohol or acetone to precipitate the calcium ascorbate. Instead, the entire process is carried out in purified water, and the calcium ascorbate is recovered by over-drying the mixture. Problems encountered early on in obtaining uniform consistency prompted owners Gerald Elders and Dick Markham to institute strict quality control standards. Over the next several years, many noted experts encompassing the diverse fields of analytical (Drs. William Peterson and Howard Jordi) and organic (Dr. Seth Rose) chemistry, nutrition (Dr. Jeffrey Bland) and biochemistry (Dr. Anthony Verlangieri) were engaged to unravel the complex makeup of Ester-C.

Extensive analyses of the ascorbate revealed anomalies in its properties, compared to those of calcium ascorbate; analytical investigations, discussions and voluminous scientific correspondence among the collaborating scientists prompted a working definition of this product as a *polyascorbate*—i.e., calcium ascorbate plus C metabolites or else a polymerized form of calcium ascorbate. The name Ester-C, was prompted by the inital deduction that the product was a polymer of calcium ascorbate in an ester linkage. Today Ester-C is regarded as a tradename, not a descriptive name, even though ascorbic acid's structure could be viewed as an ester.

Subsequent research, which is now pointing the way to a novel, exciting facet of vitamin C research, has revealed that Ester-C ascorbate is actually a mixture of calcium ascorbate, dehydroascorbic acid, aldonic acids (C metabolites), unreacted calcium carbonate and water, and a small amount of lecithin. The initial discovery that metabolites are actually a constituent of Ester-C ascorbate is a classic scientific serendipity story, told to me in 1989 by Dr. Seth Rose, the organic chemist who identified a metabolite as part of Ester-C back in 1986.

Dr. Howard Jordi, using the technique of high pressure liquid chromatography (HPLC), had enriched a fraction of Ester-C ascorbate, which he presumed was the high molecular weight polyascorbate fraction. Dr. Rose isolated the exclusion volume of the sample, which he hypothesized was the active fraction of the presumed polymeric polyascorbate, and subjected this sample to analysis by nuclear magnetic resonance (NMR) spectroscopy. Frustrated by not being able, no matter how long he tried, to fit the NMR results with a polymeric polyascorbate structure, he started to doodle on a piece of scrap paper what the proposed structure of the NMR analysis would be, without prejudice or reference to his preconceived hypothesis. He realized that the 4-carbon structure he had drawn actually represented a metabolite product, an aldonic acid, of vitamin C. (See Fig. 3.) Next, in accordance with standard scientific procedure, he had to prepare authentic aldonic acids, match them with the substances identified from Howard Jordi's fraction, and then look for these substances in Ester-C ascorbate. As usual, the inspiration came in a flash, and the rigorous proof entailed long, hard, tedious work.

Since those early days, considerable research on

cells, animals and humans has been initiated with metabolite substances of vitamin C[37,67,207]. This is definitely an area of research that will rewrite our current biochemical understanding of vitamin C metabolism, which could still be termed, despite the thousands of published papers, primitive.

Ester-C Ascorbate: Superior Absorption and Retention

It is highly unusual for a patent to be issued on a novel form of a vitamin. Yet, because of the unique properties of Ester-C ascorbate, the Commissioner of Patents and Trademarks of the United States issued Patent No. 4,822,816 to this substance on April 18, 1989[146]. Worldwide patents have been applied for and are expected to be issued in the near future. The patent relates to

> an improved form of vitamin C ... improved methods for establishing vitamin C levels in the human body ... methods for improving the human body tolerance to vitamin C ... more effectively absorbed and retained in the human body ... metabolites of ascorbic acid ... corresponding to three specific aldonic acids: L-threonic acid, L-xylonic acid and L-lyxonic acid.

The clinical data from both animal and human studies demonstrate that Ester-C ascorbate, this mixture of calcium ascorbate with natural metabolites, is in fact absorbed at a higher rate and excreted at a lower rate than both ascorbic acid (Fig. 9, Appendix) and calcium ascorbate[37,226-29,241]. See the Appendix for a more detailed discussion of the contrasts between Ester-C and other forms of vitamin C.

Vitamin C: The Master Nutrient

Studies performed by Dr. Verlangieri's group comparing the absorption in rats of Ester-C ascorbate relative to ascorbic acid[225] and calcium ascorbate[228] had the following results:

1. Ester-C was absorbed within twenty minutes, ascorbic acid only after 40 minutes[225].

2. The absorption rate for Ester-C, compared to that for ascorbic acid, was more than double. (See Fig. 9, Appendix.) The statistical significance of this value is extremely high[225]. The absorption rate of Ester-C was also double that of calcium ascorbate, 0.04 μg/ min, compared to 0.02 μg/min[228].

3. Blood plasma concentrations of vitamin C were higher in Ester-C treated animals at 20, 40 and 80 minutes[225].

4. The excretion rate of Ester-C was slower than that of ascorbic acid[225].

5. In experiments designed to assess the effects of metabolites on vitamin C absorption, the absorption of calcium ascorbate "spiked" with the metabolite calcium threonate, exceeded that of plain calcium ascorbate, and equalled or slightly exceeded that of Ester-C[226-27].

The Future of Metabolites and Ester-C Ascorbate

This clinical evidence documents the potentiating effects of metabolites on the absorption and retention of vitamin C. In fact, simply "spiking" ordinary calcium ascorbate with a metabolite makes it behave as if it were Ester-C ascorbate[226-27], which is a mixture of vitamin C and metabolites. And, as we have seen in Chapter 10, metabolites may have a role in vitamin C's inhibitory effect on HIV infection. The biochemical and pharmacological bases for the effects of metabolites on vitamin C action may open an entirely new research vista, investigating the molecular mechanisms of these small, simple molecules, metabolites.

How Do Vitamin C and Metabolites Work?

How far have we actually come in our knowledge and understanding of what vitamin C is and how it works? Although this may seem an impertinent question in the light of the massive stacks of research published on the subject, it is important to bear in mind that the essential definition of vitamin C (vitamin or essential nutrient), its therapeutic role in treating illness, and optimal human nutritional requirements are all issues considered controversial by some members of the medical and orthomolecular professions[122,138,140,150]. This is apart from considerations of the efficacy of its different forms, and indeed the biochemical and pharmacological modes of action of vitamin C's metabolites[107], which until very recently had been formulæ confined to schematics of metabolic pathways of vitamin C. The discovery of the modulating roles of metabolites and their biochemical isolation will almost certainly rewrite all our textbooks to make room for the treatment of vitamin C's many physiological and hormonal roles in the body.

Today, some 250 years after citrus fruit was identified as a preventative for scurvy, and some 60 years after the actual isolation of vitamin C[202], it is vital to review progress made in our understanding of what vitamin C is and how it works[138]. Table 4 below reviews some of the major fundamental processes identified to date in which vitamin C is intimately and essentially involved and/or required.

97

Vitamin C: The Master Nutrient

Table 4. Functional Metabolic Rates of Vitamin C

Process	Functions _____
Collagen synthesis[52,54,166,200]	Creation, maintenance of structural integrity of skin, muscle, bone, gums, all connective tissues; wound healing
Hormone and neurotransmitter synthesis[68,72,89,101,136,137,139]	Neurochemical and endocrine functions in pituitary, pancreas, gonads, thyroid, hypothalamus; production and protection of c-AMP and c-GMP
Antioxidant, vitamin E regenerator[7,33,65,101,112,161,182]	Neutralize extracellularly reactive oxidants, protect against free radical and lipid peroxidation damage
Sugar metabolism modulator[167,221,223]	Interaction with insulin and glucose in regulation of sugar homeostasis
Fat metabolism regulator[82-88,109,135]	Regulation of cholesterol levels, fatty acid metabolism, prostaglandin synthesis, L-carnitine synthesis
Modulator of oxygen-hemoglobin dissociation curve[138]	Regulates blood oxygen levels
Antiviral activity in AIDS and cancer[43,60,97,158,166]	Immune, free radical, metabolite action
Modulator of drug metabolism[24-27,173,192,210,245]	Free radical, metabolite(?) action

How Does Vitamin C Work?

When we look at Table 4 and recall that vitamin C is involved in hundreds of metabolic reactions in the body, the reasons behind its wide-ranging therapeutic actions become clearer and less "miraculous."

As an essential nutrient, required for the synthesis of other vital nutrients such as collagen and L-carnitine, as a free radical scavenger which protects against membrane and cellular damage from toxic oxygen species, as an immune enhancer strengthening our resistance to attack by other organisms, as well as neuroendrocrinal synthesis, it is no wonder that vitamin C has such pervasive therapeutic effects when administered in optimal doses.

Some of these functions are accomplished through the vitamin's outstanding capacity to be both an electron donor and electron acceptor, which accounts for its multifarious participation in numerous biochemical hydroxylations, antioxidant and free-radical scavenger regenerating abilities. This antioxidant role is doubtless the reason for the high concentration of vitamin C in neutrophils, which use superoxide to destroy foreign invaders. These toxic oxygen species are neutralized by free radical scavengers such as vitamin C.

The requirement for vitamin C in so many metabolic processes really speaks of its ubiquity prior to the hypothesized evolutionary accident that prevented humans from synthesizing their own vitamin C.

In reviewing the sorry state of our environment, the magnitude of stresses prevalent in our lives, the poor nutritional quality of our food and the excesses in our diets, it is clear from many epidemiological studies that perhaps a majority of people suffer from deficiencies of vitamin C and doubtless other nutrients as well. In light of such cellular deficiencies of vitamin C, it is not surprising that small doses may just not be adequate to "boost" the systems depleted of this nutrient.

To illustrate how stress on our immune system can deplete body stores of vitamin C, we can turn to some remarkable research conducted by MIT biologist Susumu Tonegawa, who was awarded the Nobel Prize in 1987 for his unraveling of the complex process whereby B-cells, the body's antibody-producing cells, can generate millions or billions of different antibodies, not by using a different gene for each antibody, but by shuffling and combining different portions of about a thousand genes. Early in 1990, researchers at the Whitehead Institute announced the discovery of the recombination activating gene (RAG-1) necessary to this combining process. As stress to the immune system causes the production of antibodies, and the process of antibody production requires vitamins A and C and zinc, it is clear that such stress results in the depletion of these nutrients, particularly vitamin C. And, as mentioned above, about half of us start with a lowered supply of vitamin C.

The recent announcement of new Recommended Dietary Allowances (RDAs) by the National Research Council, unchanged at 60 mg a day for nonsmokers but increased to 100 mg a day for smokers, prompted a vigorous protest from many leading nutritional authorities. In Dr. Verlangieri's words, the NRC "has chosen to ignore worldwide studies that show that vitamin C plays a role in many conditions that include degenerative tissue diseases, cataract formation, periodontal disease, immunological disease, wound healing, anemia, atherosclerosis and free radical scavenging." Why the medical and scientific research establishments continue to view vitamin C as being required in exceedingly small doses merely to prevent scurvy, despite such clinical and research evidence documenting its therapeutic potency in high doses, defies the understanding of the author, and underscores the importance of improving communication among the health professions.

Possible Functions of Vitamin C Metabolites

Thus far, based on the results of experiments described throughout this work, the known effects of metabolites on vitamin C utilization are to:

1. Increase the rate of absorption of vitamin C.

2. Increase the amount of time that vitamin C is retained in the body prior to excretion.

3. Increase the delivery of vitamin C to tissues, to enable it to achieve its therapeutic effects. This would presumably occur during the "extra" time that vitamin C is circulating in the body.

4. Enhance vitamin C's antiviral effects, as postulated with the AIDS virus and in cancer patients. This activity is as yet only speculatively attributed to the action of metabolites.

Ability to Modulate Metabolism

These effects of metabolites on vitamin C metabolism bear a strong resemblance to the way that vitamin C can exert a potentiating effect on drugs and other substances, including insulin. (See Chapter 6.) Even as far back as 1941, Richards et al.[173] described how vitamin C deficiency decreased drug (pentobarbital) oxidation and prolonged sleeping times in scorbutic guinea pigs, which would be reversed by supplementation. Also, vitamin C enhances the ability of young animals to eliminate caffeine, another drug[25,210]. Since vitamin C increases the rate of conversion of dopamine to norepinephrine[140] and thus modulates neuroendocrine levels in many endocrine tissues (pituitary, pancreas, gonads, thyroid, hypothalamus), it is easily seen how vitamin C and possibly its metabolites could modulate the utilization of many metabolic compounds and drugs.

It is also clear from experiments described previously that metabolites added to calcium ascorbate actually potentiated its absorption and retention time, equalling or exceeding the action of Ester-C ascorbate, which contains natural metabolites[226-27]. Also, as discussed in Chapter 3, prolonged exposure of HIV-infected cells to ascorbic acid resulted in 99 percent inhibition of reverse transcriptase activity and other HIV parameters (See Fig. 6–8, Appendix.), although vitamin C had no direct effect upon HIV[97].

These pioneering experiments may point the way to how metabolites work. It is possible that these modulating effects of metabolites are due to:

1. Structural (stereospecific) qualities of metabolites that interact with membranes in certain ways to enhance action of vitamin C.

2. The oxidation of vitamin C, which gives rise to metabolites and perhaps exerts antiviral effects.

3. Either or both of the above, and yet-to-be-discovered mechanisms of metabolites.

Questions That Need Answers

It would appear that, despite considerable clinical experience with vitamin C, we are still at a very primitive level of understanding of its mode of action or that of its metabolites. Certain basic questions which, if addressed, could shed light and advance our knowledge of this multifaceted nutrient, are:

1. Definition, classification and nomenclature of metabolites. In the metabolic pathway of vitamin C, which molecules are considered metabolites? Is dehydroascorbic acid a metabolite? Diketogulonic acid, etc.?

2. More precise scheme for vitamin C, including the fate of metabolites during absorption, retention and elimination from the body.

3. Is it vitamin C itself, its metabolites, or the combination of the two, that exerts the many therapeutic properties discussed throughout this book?

4. How does vitamin C exert its antiviral and anticancer effects, and what is the role of metabolites?

Chapter 12

HOW MUCH DO YOU NEED?

The Dosage Controversy

There is an extreme difference between the 60 *milligram* per day Recommended Dietary Allowance (RDA)[179]—100 mg for smokers—and the 10, 20 or more *grams* of vitamin C suggested for the therapeutic treatment of various illnesses[46]. The very low RDAs are the amounts of vitamin C that have been shown to prevent overt scurvy, and without this minimal amount of it, humans will die.

It is very difficult to measure our state of health, because it is in constant fluctuation in terms of several parameters: exposure to pathogens such as viruses and bacteria; exposure to allergens; physical and emotional stresses; and dietary abuse—e.g., too much sugar, caffeine or alcohol. Also, our emotional and psychological sense of well-being affects very many of the body's metabolic processes.

How Much Do You Need?

The myth that almost everybody believes, even in the face of extensive clinical evidence to the contrary, is that the body can store only a limited amount of vitamin C, and that it is therefore a waste of money to take any more than this amount, as it will only be excreted in the urine. The truth is that our bodily reserves of vitamin C fluctuate according to how much is needed to buttress the immune system, scavenge free radicals, regulate cholesterol and sugar metabolism, repair wounds, etc.

According to Dr. Robert Cathcart, a well-nourished person would normally have a body store of more than 5 grams of vitamin C[46]. Most individuals' vitamin C supplies are far below this level, placing them, Dr. Cathcart notes, at substantial "risk for many problems related to failure of metabolic processes dependent upon ascorbate," In fact, the list of problems Dr. Cathcart suggests may be exacerbated by severe depletion of ascorbate is considerable:

immune disorders
rheumatoid arthritis
allergic reactions
chronic infections
scarlet fever
blood coagulation
    processes
heart and blood pressure
    conditions

stress-coping mechanisms
    of the adrenals
impaired wound healing
    of bed sores, hernias,
    etc.
spinal disc degeneration
nervous-system and
    psychiatric disorders
cancers

Thus, in an optimal state of health, lack of stress and so on, an individual's bodily requirement for vitamin C could be in balance with his dietary and supplementary intake. However, if he suffered from hay fever and was exposed to ragweed, or came down with a nasty cold, his immune system would require many times more vitamin C in order to restore good health. In other words, when under severe stress, the body can "soak up" great quantities of vitamin C which at other times it would not need.

While it is clear that there can be no hard and fast rule about exactly how much vitamin C to take for your particular momentary state of health, Drs. Linus Pauling[166], Emanuel Cheraskin[54] and others give approximate guidelines in advising the intake of 1 to 3 grams per day, but the absolute best way to know how much vitamin C you need is to *ask your body*.

This is what the "bowel tolerance technique" is about: titrating your individual body chemistry at any one time to ascertain how much vitamin C you need. This method was developed by Dr. Robert Cathcart[46], who has extensive experience—more than 13,000 patients—with vitamin C, and who has used it to treat a large list of conditions including colds, hepatitis, mononucleosis, cancer and AIDS.

The Bowel Tolerance Technique

This method takes advantage of the body's way of showing you when you have taken enough vitamin C—diarrhea occurs. This is because the presence of a concentrated solution of a substance—in this case vitamin C—in the intestinal cells pulls water in from the surrounding cells, loosing the stool and producing diarrhea[28]. Diarrhea occurs only in response to the excess vitamin C that reaches the intestines and is not absorbed by the body[46]. In other words, when you have exceeded the level of vitamin C that you need at that moment, your body lets you know this by producing diarrhea. The optimum level of vitamin C to take is therefore just short of this bowel tolerance, or diarrhea-causing, level.

Your body's bowel tolerance will shift dramatically, depending on how stressed your body is. It may range from 1 gram or less when you are perfectly healthy to 20 or even 50 g when you have a very bad cold or influenza, or even 150 to 200 g for mononucleosis. It would be difficult to take 200 g orally; these high doses are achieved with a mixture of oral and intravenous administration by a physician. Table 5 lists various conditions and the therapeutic vitamin C dosage recommended by Dr. Cathcart.

Table 5. Usual Bowel Tolerance Doses.

Condition	Grams vitamin C per 24 hours	No. of doses per 24 hours
Normal	4-15	4
Mild cold	30-60	6-10
Severe cold	60-100	8-15
Influenza	100-150	8-20
ECHO, Coxsackie virus	100-150	8-20
Mononucleosis	150-200	12-25
Viral pneumonia	100-200	12-25
Hay fever, asthma	15-50	4-8
Environmental and food allergy	0.5-50	4-8
Burn, injury, surgery	25-150	6-20
Anxiety, exercise, mild stresses	15-25	4-6
Cancer	15-200	4-15
Ankylosing spondylitis	15-200	4-15
Reiter's syndrome	15-60	4-10

Vitamin C: The Master Nutrient

Condition	Grams vitamin C per 24 hours	No. of doses per 24 hours
Acute anterior uveitis	30-100	4-15
Rheumatoid arthritis	15-100	4-15
Bacterial infections	30-200	10-25
Infectious hepatitis	30-100	6-15
Candida infections	15-200	6-25

From Cathcart, R., "Vitamin C, titrating to bowel tolerance, anascorbemia and acute induced scurvy." *Medical Hypotheses* 7:1359-76, 1981[46].

How to Achieve Bowel Tolerance

Bowel tolerance level is that at which "maximum relief of symptoms which can be expected with oral doses of ascorbic acid is obtained at a point just short of the amount which produces diarrhea"[46]. Dr. Cathcart notes that effect upon acute symptoms does not occur until doses of 80 to 90 percent of bowel tolerance are reached. This means that if you take less vitamin C than the amount your body actually needs, you may not notice dramatic—or perhaps any— effects on your symptoms. The small doses prescribed in many clinical trials with colds did exert some effect, but probably not the optimal effect that could have been achieved with subjects pushed to bowel tolerance.

It is relatively easy to determine your own bowel tolerance level. You may need to start gradually and build up to this level. Many people can absorb up to 10 grams of vitamin C without diarrhea; others have diarrhea with only 1 g. Start taking 1 to 2 g vitamin C 3 times a day, for a total daily dose of 3 to 6 g. After a week, slowly increase this amount to 4 daily doses, then 5, until you reach the point at which cramps and loose stools occur. This will be very easy to notice. The amount that you have taken represents your bowel tolerance of vitamin C at that specific time. It is important to take vitamin C regularly throughout the day, at least 3 times daily. When you are ill, it may be necessary to take 1 to 2 g each hour to experience relief. With some experience, you will come to know instinctively how much vitamin C to take, somewhere between the amount that makes you feel good and the amount that causes diarrhea. And you will surely notice that this level will rise dramatically when you are sick, and return to normal when you are well. Taking vitamin C to bowel tolerance level will mean that you will always be giving your body its optimum requirement of this vital nutrient.

The majority of people, perhaps 80 to 85 percent, tolerate vitamin C without any difficulties, but a significant minority do suffer gastrointestinal upsets, including gas and diarrhea. It should be borne in mind that often the underlying problem with such gastric upsets is an imbalance in the ecology of the internal flora, especially the overgrowth of organisms such as *Candida albicans*. Attention to, and restoration of, the correct balance of intestinal flora will often enhance many aspects of health, not merely tolerance to vitamin C.

The producers of buffered mineral ascorbates, including Ester-C ascorbate, claim that one advantage of their form of vitamin C is that it produces less stomach and intestinal upset than ascorbic acid due to the buffering. The acidity of vitamin C in the intestines, where absorption occurs, irritates the mucous membranes and causes the vitamin to be expelled rapidly. Buffered vitamin C does not produce this effect, although it does produce CO_2 gas. Ester-C ascorbate does not produce CO_2, since it has been bonded and prereacted during its synthesis.

Dr. Cathcart uses ascorbic acid, rather than buffered vitamin C, initially in crystals rather than capsules, because he feels it has a stronger "punch"[49]. Once experienced with crystals, patients graduate to capsules or tablets. Other physicians prefer buffered ascorbates such as Ester-C ascorbate because of these digestive attributes. We are all biochemically unique and individual, so that each person can, after trying various forms of vitamin C, usually determine which suits him or her best.

If you are persuaded by the evidence that vitamin C can affect your health positively, you owe it to yourself to experience the optimum effect, which means going all the way to bowel tolerance levels.

Other Methods of Determining Vitamin C Levels

Urine C-Strips. There are a number of commercially available test papers which can provide a good approximation of the level of your urinary vitamin C concentration. With one of these—e.g, Wholesale Nutrition's C-Strips—vitamin C turns the blue strips white. The number of seconds it takes for the strip to turn white indicates the concentration of urinary vitamin C, with the help of the tables provided. The package includes guidelines indicating optimum, borderline and "sick" ranges of vitamin C urinary levels.

Urinary excretion levels are subject to considerable variation, and so are recommended as an approximate rather than a precise measure of body vitamin C levels[54]. They are a most important alarm indicator if they indicate *no* detectable vitamin C in the urine. This indicates that your body reserve of vitamin C has been seriously depleted, and should be replenished immediately to afford you maximum health protection.

Laboratory tests to measure plasma and leukocyte vitamin C levels. A reliable yet convenient indicator of vitamin C levels is still being sought[134]. Plasma[96] is considered to indicate metabolic turnover status of vitamin C, while leukocyte concentrations arc thought to provide a better measure of tissue stores of vitamin C. However, vitamin C utilization differs even within the different types of leukocyte cells (mononuclear and polymorphonuclear), and there is no easy or reliable correlation between plasma and leukocyte vitamin C levels[26]. It is more technically difficult to prepare these different leukocyte fractions than simply to assess plasma. Applications of techniques such as high-performance liquid chromatograpy (HPLC)[19,162] will doubtless accelerate the development of a simple, easy and reliable test of vitamin C concentration.

Intradermal test. This somewhat painful, inconvenient and time-consuming procedure has also been used to measure tissue levels of vitamin C. It involves injecting dye solution to produce a weal on the forearm and timing how long it takes for it to become completely decolorized. Twenty minutes or less is a good result; from 20 to 30 minutes is borderline; longer than 30 minutes is unacceptable[54]. Not exactly the most user-friendly do-it-yourself technique, and recommended only for those who enjoy sticking themselves with needles.

Lingual ascorbic acid test (LAAT). This is a much more palatable method of measuring vitamin C status. A drop (from a 2 gauge needle) of blue dye (2.6 dichloroindophenol sodium salt solution) is dropped onto the tip of the tongue. The time it takes for the dye to disappear indicates vitamin C status: less than 20 seconds is good; 20 to 25 seconds, marginal; longer than 25 seconds represents depletion of vitamin C levels.

Chapter 13

VITAMIN C AND OPTIMAL HEALTH

Who is not interested in achieving the *optimum* in every aspect of their life and those of their loved ones? It is difficult to imagine that anyone would choose ill-health, disease and suffering rather than vibrant health, happiness and prosperity. Given the unique determinants of who we are and what our specific situation is, what can we do to create what we really want in all aspects of our lives? The answer goes far beyond any single component—diet, supplements, subtle energies, exercise, spirituality—and yet must embrace an individually determined synergistic totality of all these elements.

Despite the multitude of advertising claims emanating from a seemingly limitless array of products, services and psychological and spiritual programs, the magical answer to whatever you want in your life is not the latest vitamin or mineral discovery that comes in a bottle, or the newest form of spiritual awareness practice, or the most sophisticated regimen of food abstinence or combining. Any or all of these may be instrumental or essential to your goal, but in the final analysis it is *you* who plans, decides and follows your own life path.

Each of us is unique in so many ways—genetically, metabolically, nutritionally, emotionally, spiritually—that the combination of food and lifestyle that works for a Norman Cousins[59] or a Louise Hay[100] will not necessarily work for you. And the proof of the wisdom of these and many more individuals, including authors Cheraskin[54] and Pauling[166], is that they emphatically recommend that each person discover and develop what works for him or her. There are general guidelines on diet, supplements and exercise that are a good starting place. This book has considered in great deal many of the therapeutic aspects of vitamin C, one invaluable component of almost any health- and life-enhancing regime. This chapter will consider some of the other vital ingredients and practices that together might constitute and/or supplement your personal program for attaining optimal well-being.

Attitude Toward Health and Practitioners

Your role in your health program is crucial. Are you simply the body that gets sick, and the doctor the one who heals you? Do you follow your doctor's orders religiously without even questioning what he is prescribing for you? Do you know the potential side effects of medications you are taking and what would happen if you didn't take them? Do you participate in formulating your own health care regime?

Do you exercise the same degree of consumer awareness, common sense and discrimination in choosing your practitioner as you do in buying a carpet or stereo, or even in considering the color and design of new wallpaper?

It is truly shocking that many people place themselves totally in the hands of their doctors and completely abdicate responsibility for their own health. There is a belief that doctors, by virtue of their training, know everything about everyone. The idea of questioning or even having a conversation about any proposed treatment with one's doctor is considered almost heresy. Yet doctors are the first to admit that they are fallible, human, overworked, do not have time to look into many contributory aspects of illness, and are not generally trained in nutrition, counseling, bereavement, etc.

What do we expect of doctors? They have not lived in our bodies. Doctors generally are well-trained and technically proficient within their particular specialty. The best physicians are also superbly humane, compassionate and empathetic, and realize that the efficacy of their medicine depends to a large degree on the patient's state of mind, will to live and other intangible qualities.

One of the most important components in your health program is your choice of a health practitioner or practitioners. The choice could vary enormously, from a single general practitioner or orthomolecular physician to a team of complementary therapists you call on as and when required. It is wise to build a good support network in all aspects of your life— including health.

Vitamin C: The Master Nutrient

The paradigm of health care that appears optimal to me would place the individual at the center of a circle, surrounded by the entire range of health options available, including sophisticated 20th-century technology, traditional herbs, nutritional and botanical medicine, acupuncture, homeopathy, counseling and spiritual healing. The most appropriate therapies would be arrived at by a matching of the components of the therapies with the individual's condition. The day is eagerly awaited when consultations from across health disciplines can cross-fertilize and optimize the course of treatment for the individual concerned, who might choose to take vitamin C, homeopathic remedies and healing to counterbalance the trauma of a serious operation.

Your health program ought to include several elements: nutritious diet[234], supplements as needed, exercise, relaxation. At times, when stressed, you might need additional therapeutic support: massage, chiropractic, acupuncture, homeopathy, counseling, aromatherapy. *You* are at the center of your life. Only you can make the decisions about what therapy and which therapist to choose. And, though personal recommendations may be invaluable, only you can determine, perhaps with difficulty, whether what you are choosing is working. Except in cases of dire illness, we can usually choose another option. If we are "terminally" ill, we can still make decisions that affect the quality of the remainder of our lives, and strive to make peace with ourselves and feel gratitude for the many blessings we have experienced. To be realistic, in one sense we are all terminal, and to live each day of our lives with this recognition would benefit the planet immeasurably. The following health practice information is put forward for your consideration, contemplation and, if you see fit, your consumption. None of it should be regarded as rigid, merely as guidelines.

General Dietary Guidelines

There is a multitude of diets, each of which espouses a particular way of considering, preparing and eating food[135]. These range from the high-carbohydrate, low-protein, low-fat Pritikin diet, the raw-food Gerson cancer diet, the brown-rice-and-vegetable, yin/yang balanced macrobiotic cancer diet, all vegetarian in emphasis, to simple low-calorie "starvation" diets. What you eat represents a lot more than simply calories or biochemical nutrients—it constitutes the nuts and bolts that build your body. The old computer adage "garbage in, garbage out" applies also to the food you eat. Its quality and freshness will do more than quiet your hunger pangs, reverberating in the subtle levels of your being and providing the sustenance to build and maintain a strong, healthy body.

Here are a series of sensible dietary guidelines which can be used to enhance your health and your happiness:

1. Eat a wide variety of food that you enjoy, especially fruits, vegetables, nuts and grains. Buy produce that is free of pesticides and other toxic chemicals.

2. Prepare food in ways that do not deplete them of nutrients. Steam vegetables or eat them raw.

3. Eat more fish and chicken than red meats.

4. Eat butter rather than margarine; use virgin and cold-pressed oils for salads and frying.

5. Drastically reduce consumption of sugar, coffee and alcohol, or avoid them altogether. Do not smoke.

6. Discover your particular food allergies and avoid those foods.

7. Enjoy and celebrate food, present your meals in an aesthetically pleasing manner, and eat with appreciation and gratitude.

Supplements

There seem to be two extreme all-or-nothing views on supplementation:

1. Take every vitamin, mineral and amino acid in creation—the more the merrier, and in particular combination formulae.

2. No supplements—get all nutrients from food.

Somewhere between these extremes probably lies the sensible answer for most people. In an ideal world, with pristine water and environment, stress-free, we *could* perhaps obtain what we need from our food. However, as we all know, our world is far from ideal—our water and air are fouled with polluting toxic chemicals, and our soil is depleted of vital minerals and nutrients. The prepared food we buy is refined and processed out of most of its nutritional value. The jobs we have and the lifestyles we create produce health-destroying stress, contributing to further deterioration of our health. Fascinating research is revealing how our state of mind can influence almost every organ system in the body. Even parameters of how we utilize vitamin C can apparently be modulated by our state of mind. For example, Dr. Russell Jaffe recounted to the author the finding that the half-life of vitamin C is four days rather than four hours in his friend, a 108-year-old Buddhist monk.

The following are merely guidelines for supplement use. Explore and validate your personal supplement regime with an orthomolecular physician. Because of the complex interactions among the various vitamins and minerals, it is important to know extremely well what nutrients you ought to take at any particular time. Also, as your condition changes, you may want to vary your supplement program.

Vitamins.

Vitamin A (or beta-carotene)	25,000 International Units
Vitamin B complex	25-50 milligrams
Vitamin C	3-6 grams
Vitamin E	500-1000 I.U.

(Note that the most effective form of vitamin E is the unesterified mixed tocopherol concentrate. Esterified, d- alpha tocopheryl acetate or synthetic dl forms of vitamin E are not fully effective as antioxidants.)

Minerals. Take a balanced multimineral supplement, including macro and trace minerals, including 25 to 50 mg of zinc.

Essential fatty acids. Take an EFA supplement containing linoleic and linolenic acids, also evening primrose oil and fish oils.

Vitamin C: The Master Nutrient

Other useful substances as required.

Amino acids	Bach flower remedies
Ginseng	Homeopathic remedies
Royal jelly	Essential oils
Western and Chinese herbs	

Exercise

To view exercise as a mere activity to burn off calories or keep your cardiovascular system fit is short-changing yourself. With the entire spectrum of recreational activities available, it should be possible to choose activities you genuinely relish, and go at them with gusto. Whether it be dancing, walking, golf, tennis, skiing or trampoline bouncing to music, enjoyment is a bonus that significantly benefits both health and psyche. Exercise, in addition to its cardiovascular benefits, strengthens the immune system and releases beneficial neurohormones which aid in relaxation.

Walking, especially while taking deep breaths, is a time- honored tonic for mind, body and spirit. While certain individuals may crave and even require the physical exhaustion that marathon runs engender, every person is unique. Exercises such as walking, yoga and Tai Chi can be combined with relaxation and meditation practices to enhance the beneficial effects on health.

Emotional and Spiritual Well-Being

How we feel about ourselves, our self-esteem, our ability to cope with daily living situations—these have a tremendous influence upon our health, our happiness, even our financial prosperity. The medical literature abounds in correlations between the stresses of lifestyle changes, divorce and bereavement and detrimental effects on our health. Profiles of Type A personalities being more prone to heart attacks, the assessment of personality profiles for other diseases such as cancer, and even the esoteric causes of illness, are being compiled[100]. Norman Cousins in his book *The Healing Heart*[59] graphically describes how overwhelming feelings of panic can occur when even someone like himself, an expert in positive mental attitude, is faced with a life-threatening illness.

On a practical level, what can we do when we get angry, frustrated or devastated? Very often the people who need to cry the most are those who are unable to, those who need to vent their anger insist they are never angry, or the people who are loneliest retreat deeper and deeper into solitude. Our feelings and aspirations are an integral part of who we are, and to disown or disavow them is to kill a beautiful component of our life. Expressing our rage in ways that don't harm others, sharing our vulnerability and hopelessness, finding the courage to be ourselves—these are practices that certainly will be reflected in greater health and happiness.

Vitamin C and Ester-C Ascorbate Compared

The marketplace contains a variety of forms of vitamin C: plain ascorbic acid in crystals, tablets, capsules or timed-release capsules; mineral ascorbates (sodium and calcium ascorbate); food or "natural" sources of vitamin C (sago palm, rose hips acerola, beet, citrus). Once inside the body's biochemical factory, these are all the same substance—vitamin C. Experts like Linus Pauling and Robert Cathcart have been maintaining this for years, yet some consumers are being persuaded to pay significantly more for "natural source" vitamin C. There is a difference with Ester-C ascorbate because Ester-C is the only form of vitamin C that has included naturally-occurring, body-ready metabolites, which enhance and potentize the effects of vitamin C.

The pharmaceutical promise of these metabolites is only beginning to be realized. It is quite possible that in the future we will be able to purchase metabolites which will have modulating effects on other substances than vitamin C.

Another difference between Ester-C and all other vitamin C products is that, while vitamin C and the mineral ascorbates are water-soluble, Ester-C is fat-soluble as well. As mentioned in Chapter 5, this may in fact enhance the regeneration of membrane-bound vitamin E, although research has yet to be done on this matter. Although Ester-C is apparently not stored in the fat, research is needed to establish that this is in fact the case.

Seeing More Clearly: Vitamin C and Cataracts

Recent biochemical and epidemiological research reveals that vitamin C may be a significant protective factor in preventing cataract formation and in promoting healthy eye tissues[141]. Ascorbic acid levels are high in ocular tissues, and vitamin C has been postulated to act as a protector against oxidation and free-radical damage. In fact, with a progressing cataract, vitamin C levels decline, not from a reduction in the supply of ascorbic acid but due to a rapid oxidation of vitamin C.

It has been known that during autoxidation of ascorbic acid solutions, the color changes from transparent to dark brown, very much like the changes observed in lenses during cataract formation. Reports from the University of Western Ontario compared 175 cataract patients with 175 age- and sex-matched cataract-free controls. The only significant difference between the groups was their intake of vitamins E and C. Vitamin E intake was associated with a 56 percent lower cataract risk, while vitamin C intake correlated with a 70 percent lower risk, compared with those who took no vitamins. These human studies confirm results from earlier animal studies which demonstrated the protective effects of vitamin E against cataract formation in diabetic rats. Another epidemiological study showed that high levels of the antioxidants vitamins E and C and beta-carotene exerted a protective effect against cataract formation.

Thus the benefits of vitamin C may actually be visible, as well as tangible and palpable.

A Final Word About Vitamin C

For all of vitamin C's considerable therapeutic properties, it is not a panacea that will automatically cure all ills. Having said this, however, it is hard to think of any substance that is superior to vitamin C in its preventive and therapeutic properties. Here we have a safe, natural and inexpensive substance, an integral component of body systems, that manages our cholesterol levels, strengthens the immune system, builds stronger bones, modulates our hormones, reverses heart disease and kills viruses, even the deadly AIDS virus. Plain ascorbic acid, timed-release ascorbic acid, mineral ascorbates, Ester-C ascorbate—tailor your choice of vitamin C to your personal needs and experience, but don't leave home without it!

APPENDIX

This appendix further elaborates on the principles and information presented in previous chapters of this book, but in greater technical detail, for the benefit of physicians and other health professionals. Each section is keyed to the chapter in which its topic is presented in the main body of the book.

CHAPTER 3: VITAMIN C AND ESTER-C METABOLISM AND METABOLITES

Chemical formulae and biochemical pathways are not engraved as in stone upon the brains of scientists, at least not upon that of the author. Even after many years and advanced courses in biochemistry, physiology, etc., these pathways fade from memory unless in constant use. And, with the incredibly rapid advances in knowledge being made in science and medicine, much material may simply be new and not have been taught during one's formal training. These formulae are presented here as aids in understanding and as a convenient reference tool.

Structure and Biosynthesis of Vitamin C

Vitamin C, also known as L-ascorbic acid, L-xyloascorbic acid, 3-oxo-L-gulofuranolactone (enol form), L-3-ketothreonic acid lactone and antiscorbutic vitamin, has the chemical formula $C_6H_8O_6$ and a molecular weight of 176.12. This 6-carbon molecule is structurally very similar to the sugar D glucose (Fig. 1), a point of significance which will be addressed when considering the mode of action and mechanisms underlying vitamin C's therapeutic effectiveness with diabetes and heart disease.

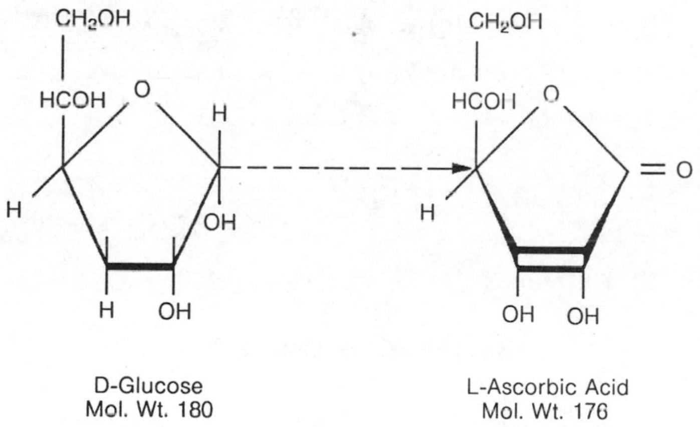

D-Glucose
Mol. Wt. 180

L-Ascorbic Acid
Mol. Wt. 176

Fig. 1
Molecular structures of D-glucose and L-ascorbic acid.

Vitamin C: The Master Nutrient

Vitamin C, found naturally throughout most of the plant and animal kingdoms, is synthesized from glucuronic or galactonic acid derived from the sugar glucose in the following biosynthetic process (Fig. 2):

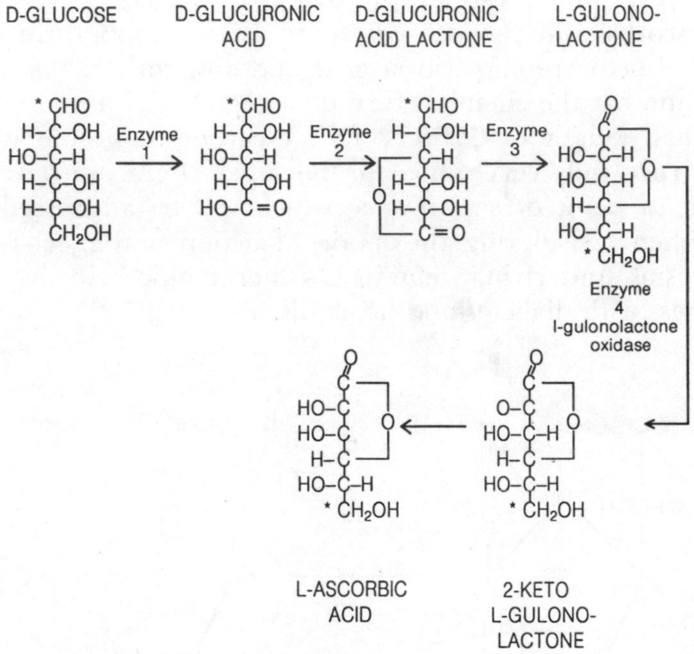

D-GLUCOSE   D-GLUCURONIC ACID   D-GLUCURONIC ACID LACTONE   L-GULONO-LACTONE

```
 * CHO          * CHO              * CHO                    O
H–C–OH  Enzyme H–C–OH   Enzyme  H–C–OH   Enzyme            C
HO–C–H    1    HO–C–H     2        C–H      3      HO–C–H
H–C–OH   ——>   H–C–OH   ——>    H–C–OH    ——>      HO–C–H   O
H–C–OH         HO–C=O          H–C–OH             H–C
 CH2OH                            C=O             HO–C–H
                                                 * CH2OH

                                                 Enzyme 4
                                                 l-gulonolactone
                                                 oxidase

             O                              O
             C                              C
HO–C                             O–C
HO–C    O    <——                HO–C–H    O
H–C                              H–C
HO–C–H                          HO–C–H
 * CH2OH                         * CH2OH

L-ASCORBIC                       2-KETO
ACID                             L-GULONO-
                                 LACTONE
```

Fig. 2
Biosynthesis of vitamin C.

As noted earlier, an evolutionary accident some 50 million years ago deprived certain species, including humans, of the enzymatic machinery for synthesizing vitamin C.

Figure 3: The Vitamin C Complex and its Degradation Products. The complete process is not fully established.

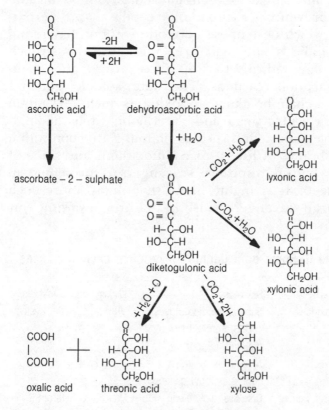

Fig. 3
Metabolism of vitamin C.

CHAPTER 5: VITAMIN C SCAVENGES POISONOUS FREE RADICALS

There are a number of natural substances, including vitamin C, which are powerful antioxidants and free radical scavengers, and which act to prevent the damaging effects of superoxides, peroxides, hydroxyl radicals and singlet oxygen molecules. These include the preventive antioxidants catalase and peroxidase which decompose peroxide without generating free radicals, and chain-breaking antioxidants which scavenge radicals to stop free radical and chain propagation reactions. The water-soluble, aqueous phase chain-breaking antioxidants include vitamin C, uric acid, cysteine and glutathione, while the lipid-soluble antioxidants such as vitamin E function within membranes. A list of toxic antioxidants and some of their known respective scavengers is presented in Table 6. It is highly likely that many more such natural scavengers exist in nature, awaiting our discovery.

Table 6. Some antioxidants for reactive oxygen species.

OXIDANTS	SCAVENGER	DIETARY ANTIOXIDANTS
Superoxide	Superoxide dismutase (SOD), ceruloplasmin, melanin, copper complexes, alpha-mercaptopriopionyl glycine	Vitamin C, rutin, cysteine
Hydrogen peroxide	Catalase, glutathione, uric acid	Vitamin C, vitamin E, selenium
Hydroxyl radical	Cholesterol, benzoate, dimethyl sulfoxide (DMSO), formate, uric acid	Vitamin C, rosemary, sage, amygdalin, anthocyanin, cysteine
Singlet oxygen	Cholesterol, bilirubin, histidine, uric acid	Vitamin E, BHT, cholesterol, lemon oil

From *Oxidology*, Bradford, Allen and Culbert, 1985. Bradford Foundation[53].

CHAPTER 6: FIGHTER OF HEART DISEASE AND DIABETES

Vitamin C Versus Heart Disease.

Vitamin C has been shown to modulate cholesterol metabolism in the following ways[83-88,157-59,193-96,215]:

1. Vitamin C increases the rate at which cholesterol is removed by its conversion to bile acids and excretion via the intestines.

2. Vitamin C increases HDL levels. High HDL levels are correlated with low risk of heart disease.

3. Vitamin C, through its laxative effect, accelerates elimination of waste, thereby acting to decrease the reabsorption of bile acids and their reconversion to cholesterol.

Clinical studies have shown that vitamin C reduces serum cholesterol and triglyceride levels in individuals with high levels. Ginter[85] showed that 1 g/day vitamin C led, after three months, to a decline in plasma cholesterol levels by 10 percent and triglycerides by 40 percent. Another study[78] showed that 3 g/day vitamin C decreased cholesterol by 18 percent and triglycerides by 12 percent after three weeks. Vitamin C does not reduce cholesterol or triglyceride levels in individuals who are within the range of "normal" values[118], suggesting that vitamin C acts in a homeostatic way to promote equilibrium.

Work by Dr. Anthony Verlangieri's group discussed in Chapter 6 has shown that sulfate groups play a critical role in supporting the strength of the GAG matrix[10,157]. High sulfate levels are correlated with low cholesterol levels; low sulfate levels with high cholesterol[220]. Removal of sulfate groups by an enzyme called aryl sulfatase B leads to degradation of the GAG matrix. Vitamin C has been shown to inhibit this enzyme and thus prevents the removal of the sulfate group of the GAG matrix[223]. These methodical and rigorous studies at the molecular level support the theory that one of the key elements in preventing and controlling atherosclerosis is the maintenance of structural integrity of cell and arterial linings. Vitamin C, involved directly in collagen synthesis and in the inhibition of aryl sulfatase B, obviously is an important factor in supporting the structural integrity of the body tissues.

Additional elegant studies, initially with rabbits[224] and more recently using noninvasive ultrasound techniques in monkeys[222], have also demonstrated that arteries with high vitamin C levels have lower cholesterol levels and that vitamins C and E can actually reverse the disease process of atherosclerosis[233]! See Fig. 4.

Average Percent Stenosis in Primate Carotid Arteries

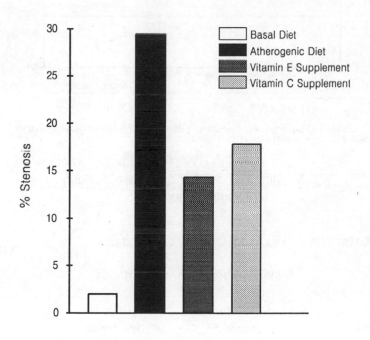

Fig. 4. Effect of vitamins E and C upon arterial stenosis (narrowing)[230].

Vitamin C: The Master Nutrient

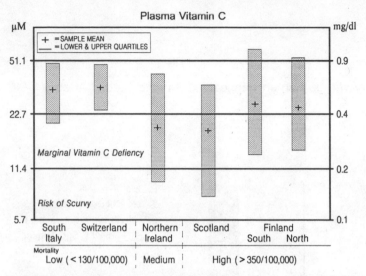

FIGURE 5. Cross-sectional comparison of plasma vitamin C in European populations with different mortality from IHD.

Fig. 5. Vitamin C and heart disease mortality in European countries[82].

CHAPTER 7: VITAMIN C AND ARTHRITIS

Table 7. Classification of Arthritis

INFECTIOUS	INFLAMMATORY	METABOLIC
Bacterial:	Rheumatoid	Osteoarthritis
Staphylococcal	Ankylosing spondylitis	Traumatic osteoporosis
Gonococcal	Juvenile rheumatoid	Aseptic necrosis
Tuberculosis	Collagen disease	Hyperparathyroidism
Streptococcus	Reiter's syndrome	Avascular necrosis
Pneumococcus	Sjögren's syndrome	

132

Appendix

Table 7. Classification of Arthritis

Parasitic:	Psoriatic	Osteoporosis
Amebic	Polymyositis	Allergic (atopic)
Malarial	Rheumatic fever	Calcium deficiency
Treponemal	Sclerodoma	Vitamin D deficiency
Viral:	Lupus erythematosus	Osteochondrosis
Hepatitis	Bechet's syndrome	Hypothyroidism
Mumps	Polychondritis	Hormonal deficiency
Rubella	Polyarteritis	Protein deficiency
Fungal:	Polymyalgia	Hypertrophic osteoarthropathy
Mycoplasmal:	Erythema nodosum	Gout

From *Fight Back Against Arthritis*, Robert B. Bingham, M.D., 1985[21].

Crippled Dogs

In another study conducted at Droruddalen Dyi-reklinikk in Oslo, Norway, Dr. Berge tested Ester-C ascorbate on 180 dogs, who were fed 3 × 30 mg/kg Ester-C ascorbate over six months. These dogs exhibited clinical symptoms of chronic joint, skeletal and muscle inflammation, which was diagnosed by journal, clinical evaluation and, in some cases, X-rays. Treatment evaluation, seven days following supplementation, after six weeks and finally after six months, was based upon clinical evaluation and owner report. One hundred dogs with the following chronic ailments were monitored in this study:

Joint injuries with secondary, permanent changes
Arthrosis
Spondylosis

Vitamin C: The Master Nutrient

Hip dysplasia

Older disc prolapse with secondary, permanent changes

Muscle atrophy as a result of functional loss

Senile wear changes in support and motion systems

The results were as follows:

Ailment		Good improvement Free of symptoms	Little improvement No effect
Hip dysplasia:	1 week	32 (71.7%)	13 (28.9%)
	6 weeks	35 (77.9%)	10 (22.2%)
Spondylosis and back prolapse:	1 week	13 (76.5%)	4 (23.5%)
	6 weeks	13 (76.5%)	4 (23.5%)
Arthrosis:	1 week	30 (78.9%)	8 (21.1%)
	6 weeks	31 (81.6%)	7 (18.4%)

The possible mechanisms for Ester-C ascorbate appearing to exert a therapeutic effect in arthritis beyond that of vitamin C^{60} are presently not fully understood. However, the case of the recovery of the dogs (which of course manufacture their own vitamin C) from their chronic ailments[73,156] in response to Ester-C supplementation is dramatic evidence that possibly the metabolites in Ester-C exert a yet-to-be-discovered powerful therapeutic effect. More rigorous further clinical trials with these dogs are presently in progress in Norway.

Excerpt from: *The Norwegian Veterinary Journal*, Vol. 102, August/September 1990, "Polyascorbate (C-Flex®) an Interesting Alternative for Problems in the Support and Movement Apparatus in Dogs." Clinical trial of Ester-C ascorbate in canines.

Appendix

CHAPTER 9: ATTACK ON VIRUSES

Table 8. Antiviral activity of vitamin C (early years)

DATE	RESEARCHER(S)	VIRUS
1935-9	Jungeblut[119–121]	Poliomyelitis
1936	Holden & Resnick[104]	Herpes
1936	Kligler & Bernkopf[130]	Vaccinia (smallpox)
1936	Lominski[143]	Bacteriophage
1937	Lngenbusch & Enderling[133]	Foot & mouth
1937	Amato[4]	Rabies
1937	Holden & Molloy[105]	Herpes
1939	Sabin[185]	Poliomyelitis
1943	Dainow[63]	Herpes (shingles)
1944	Lojkin[142]	Tobacco mosaic
1945	Paez de la Torre[163]	Measles
1949-59	Klenner[127]	Poliomyelitis
1949	Klenner[127]	Encephalitis, mumps
1950	Zureick[246]	Chicken pox
1952-54	Bauer & Staub[16,17]	Hepatitis
1963	Vargus Magne[218]	Influenza
1962	Dalton[64]	Pneumonia
1954-55	Greer[92], Gsell & Kalt[94]	Poliomyelitis

CHAPTER 10: VITAMIN C AND METABOLITES KILL THE AIDS VIRUS

Vitamin C Inhibits RT Activity and P20 Antigen, Fig. 6–7.

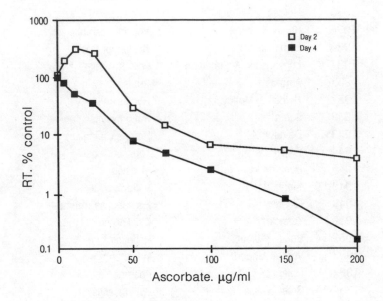

Fig. 6
Inhibition of HIV RT Activity by Vitamin C.

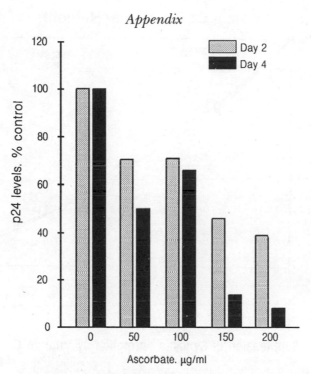

Fig. 7
Inhibition pf p24 Antigen by Vitamin C.

Vitamin C Inhibits Syncytia Formation.

A third assay of HIV infectivity involves the monitoring of giant, multicell complex formations called *syncytia*. These syncytia are formed due to the interaction of HIV cell glycoprotein with receptors on the surface of T4 cells. In non-vitamin C treated cells, syncytia became visible by day 4, reaching a peak on day 6. In contrast, with vitamin C-treated cells, syncytia were inhibited by 93.3% on day 4[97] Fig. 8, Appendix. These data are summarized in Table 9.

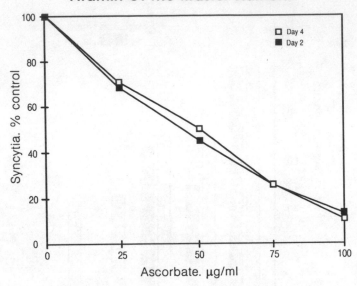

Vitamin C: The Master Nutrient

Fig. 8
Suppression of Syncytia Formation by Vitamin C.

Table 9. Inhibition of HIV activity by vitamin C

PARAMETER ASSESSED	DEGREE OF INHIBITION ATTAINED (%)
Reverse transcriptase (RT) activity	99.0
p24 antigen expression	90.0
Syncytia formation	93.9

S. Harakash and R. J. Jariwalla, 1990[97].

138

Mechanisms of Vitamin C's Inhibition of HIV

Does vitamin C act directly upon HIV, or is there some indirect process of inactivation? Experiments conducted to address this question determined that vitamin C does not directly inactivate the virus nor prevent infection of cells; however, the inhibition of HIV by vitamin C was due to vitamin C's action upon the virus, not upon other cellular processes. Since vitamin C does not by itself directly inhibit RT activity or processes involved in syncytium formation, the reduction of these viral parameters "therefore represents inhibition of a step or steps in the HIV replication . . . delayed inactivating effect on the virion-associated enzyme was seen upon prolonged incubation of cell-free virus with ascorbate. This may reflect the accumulation to threshold levels of some reactive metabolite of ascorbic acid . . . upon prolonged in vitro exposure, virion components may become susceptible to further attack by metabolites of ascorbate generated from its oxidative degradation"[97].

The actual mechanism responsible for vitamin C's anti-HIV properties is not currently known. Further research is continuing to unravel the molecular action of ascorbate on HIV.

CHAPTER 11: THE NEW SUPER C

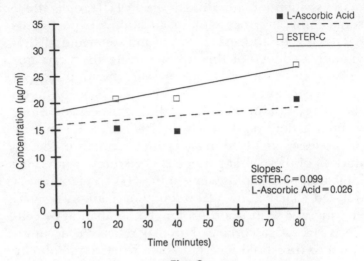

Fig. 9
**Enhanced Absorption of Ester-C compared with
L-Ascorbic Acid.**

The following is an abstract from *The FASEB Journal*, published for the 75th annual meeting of the Federation of American Societies for Experimental Biology, April 21–25, 1991.

"Effects of Calcium L-Threonate on Ascorbic Acid Uptake by Human Lymphoma Cells." M. J. Fay and A. J. Verlangieri (spon: M. C. Wilson). Dept. of Pharmacology, School of Pharmacy, University of Mississippi.

The metabolism of ascorbic acid (AA) involves the oxidation of AA to dehydroascorbic acid which subsequently undergoes a hydrolytic ring cleavage to form 2, 3-diketo-1-gulonic acid. Although much research has been done concerning the biological and pharmacological effects of AA, very little work has been done with the AA metabolites. In the present studies we investigated the effects of preincubation (1 hour) of human T-lymphoma cells with increasing concentrations of calcium L-threonate on the uptake of labled AA. The results indicate that calcium L-threonate significantly increases cellular AA uptake in a dose dependent manner, with the highest level of threonate increasing uptake approximately 177% above control levels. These results correlate with *in vivo* studies showing that Ester-C® (a calcium ascorbate supplement containing AA metabolites) is absorbed more rapidly than AA. The facilitation of cellular AA uptake and subsequent increase in celluar free radical scavaging potential may have important clinical therapeutic implications. (Supported by a fellowship to M.J. Fay from the Intercal Corp., Prescott, AZ and overhead funds from A.J. Verlangieri.)

Scurvy-Fighting Properties

The following tables and comments are excerpted from "Comparison of the Anti-Scorbutic Activity of L-Ascorbic Acid and Ester-C in the Non-Ascorbate Synthesizing Rat," a paper by Anthony J. Verlangieri, Michael J. Fay and Anthony W. Bannon published in *Life Sciences*, 48:2275-2281.

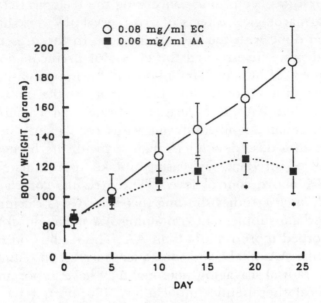

Fig. 10
Growth Curves for the AA and EC
Supplemented Rats with S.E. Bars

"It is clear from this study that, based on ascorbate activity equivalents, EC is 4 - 5x more potent or effective than AA in preventing scurvy. The authors believe, based on previous reports and from the present results, that this increase is due to calcium threonate, and possibly calcium xylonate and calcium lyxonate. Calcium threonate is present in the

142

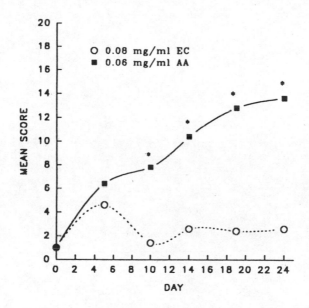

Fig. 11
Mean Total Scorbutic Ratings over Entire Study
(sum of all scores/N)

highest concentration in the EC products, and preliminary evidence suggests that it increases AA uptake in T-cells. We believe threonate facilitates cellular uptake of AA, thereby increasing its potency and immune enhancing properties compared to an equivalent ascorbate dose derived from AA."

BIBLIOGRAPHY

1. Adams, R. & Murray, F. 1978. *Improving Your Health with Vitamin C.* Larchmont.
2. Afroz, M. 1975. "Vitamins C and B$_{12}$." *Journal of the American Medical Association,* 232:3, 246.
3. Altschule, M. D. 1976. "Is It True What They Say about Cholesterol?" *Executive Health,* 12:no.11.
4. Amato, G. 1937. "Azione dell'acido ascorbico sul virus fisso della rabbia e sulla tossina tetanica." *Giornale di Batteriologia Virologia et Immunologia* (Torino), 19:843–849.
5. Anderson, J. T., Keys, A. 1957. "Safflower Oil, Hydrogenated Safflower Oil and Ascorbic Acid Effects on Serum Cholesterol in Man." Federation Proceedings (Bethesda), 16:380.
6. Anderson, R. 1982. "Effects of Ascorbate on Normal and Abnormal Leukocyte Functions, in Vitamin C: New Clinical Applications in Immunology." *Lipid Metabolism and Cancer,* ed. A. Hanck, Hans Huber, Bern, pp.23–34.
7. Anderson, R., Lukey, P. T. 1987. "A Biological Role for Ascorbate in the Selective Neutralization of Extracellular Phagocyte-derived Oxidants." In: Third Con-

ference on Vitamin C. 1987. Annals of the New York Academy of Sciences. Vol. 498.

8. Baetgen, D. "Results of the Treatment of Epidemic Hepatitis in Children with High Doses of Ascorbic Acid in the Years 1957–1958." *Medizinische Monatschrift*, 15:pp.30–36. 1961.

9. Bailer, J. C. III, E. M. 1986. "Progress Against Cancer." *New England Journal of Medicine*, 314:1226–32.

10. Baker, III E. EM. 1971. "Ascorbic Sulfate: A Urinary Metabolite of Ascorbic Acid in Man." *Science*, 173: 826–827.

11. Banerjee, S. 1944. Part IV. Effect of Vitamin C on the Insulin Content of the Pancreas of Guinea Pigs. *Annals of Bio-chemistry and Experimental Medicine*, 4:33–36.

12. Banerjee, S., Baudyopadhyay, A. 1963. Plasma Lipids in Scurvy: Effect of Ascorbic Acid Supplement and Insulin Treatment. *Proceedings* Society Experimental Biology and Medicine, 112:372–374.

13. Bartelheimer, H. 1939. "Vitamin C in the Treatment of Diabetes." *Die Medizinische Welt*, 13:117–120.

14. Bartlett, M. K., Jones, C. M., Ryan, A. E. 1942. "Vitamin C and Wound Healing. II. Ascorbic Acid Content and Tensile Strength of Healing Wounds in Human Beings." *New England Journal of Medicine*, 226:474–481.

15. Bates, C. J., Mandal, A. R., Cole, T. J. 1977. "HDL-Cholesterol and Vitamin C Status." *The Lancet*, 3:611.

16. Baur, H. 1952. "Poliomyelitis Therapy with Ascorbic Acid." *Helvetia Medica Acta*, 19:pp.470–474.

17. Baur H., Staub, H. 1954. "Therapy of Hepatitis with Ascorbic Acid Infusions." *Schweizerische Medizinische Wochenschrift*, 84:pp.595–597.

18. Becker, R. R. et al. 1953. "Ascorbic Acid Deficiency and Cholesterol Synthesis." *Journal American Chemical Society*, 75:2020.

19. Behrens, W. A., Madere, R. A Procedure for the Determination of Ascorbic and Dehydroascorbic Acid in Biological Fluids, Tissues, and Foods. In Third Conference on Vitamin C. 1987. Annals of the New York Academy of Sciences. Vol. 498.

Bibliography

20. Belfield, W. O. 1976. "Chronic Subclinical Scurvy and Canine Hip Dysplasia." *Pet Practice*. 1399– 1401. See Appendix p. 133 for related study material.
21. Bingham, R. 1984. *Fight Back Against Arthritis*. Desert Arthritis Medical Clinic.
22. Biser, S. 1989. "The Great Vitamin C Myth Exploded." *Health Discoveries Newsletter*.
23. Bjelke, E. 1974. "Epidemiological Studies of Cancer of the Stomach, Colon and Rectum with Special Emphasis on the Role of Diet." *Scan. J. Gastro.*, 9(31): 1–235.
24. Blanchard, J., Achari, R., Harrison, G. G. and Conrad, K. A. 1984. "The Influence of Vitamin C on Antipyrine Pharmacokinetics in Elderly Men." *Biopharm. & Drug Disp.*, 5: 43–54.
25. Blanchard, J., Hochman, D. 1984. "Effects of Vitamin C on Caffeine Pharmacokinetics in Young and Aged Guinea Pigs." *Drug-Nutr. Inter.*, 2:243– 55.
26. Blanchard, J., Conrad, K. A. 1988. "Comparison of Plasma, Mononuclear and Polymorphonuclear Leucocyte Vitamin C Levels in Young and Elderly Women During Depletion and Supplementation." *European Journal of Clinical Nutrition*, 43: 97–106.
27. Blanchard, J., Conrad, K. A., Mead, K. A., Gary, P. J. 1989. Vitamin C Disposition in Young and Elderly Men. Manuscript.
28. Bland, J. 1987. "The Latest Developments in the Therapy and Biochemistry of Vitamin C." Seminar Transcript.
29. Bland, J. 1989. "Reducing the Risk to Coronary Heart Disease: Appraisal of Progress." In: Nutrition, Health and Peace. Pauling Symposia. Vol. I Linus Pauling Institute. Jariwalla R. J., Schwoebel S. L. (eds).
30. Bland, J. 1989. *The Key to the Power of Vitamin C and Its Metabolites*. Keats Publishing.
31. Booker, W. M. et al. 1957. "Cholesterol–Ascorbic Acid Relationship." *American J. Phys.* 189:335–7.
32. Bordia, A. 1980. "The Effect of Vitamin C on Blood Lipids, Fibrinolytic Activity, and Platelet Adhesiveness in Patients with Coronary Artery Disease." *Atherosclerosis*, 35:2, 181–187.

147

33. Bradford, Allen & Culbert. 1985. *Oxidology*. Bradford Foundation.
34. Brandt, R., Guyer, K. E., Banks, W. L. Jr. 1974. "A Simple Method to Prevent Vitamin C Interference with Urinary Glucose Determinations." *Clinica Chimica Acta* 51:103–104.
35. Brighthope, I. 1988. *The AIDS Fighters*. Keats Publishing.
36. Burns, Rivers & Machlin (eds.). 1987. Third Conference on Vitamin C. Annals of the New York Academy of Sciences. Vol. 498.
37. Bush, M. J. & Verlangieri, A. J. 1987. "An Acute Study on the Relative Gastro-Intestinal Absorption of a Novel Form of Calcium Ascorbate." *Res. Comm. Chem. Path. Pharm.* 57 (1): 137–40.
38. Calabrese, E. J., Stoddard, A., Leonard, D. A., Dinardi, S. R. 1987. "The Effects of Vitamin C Supplementation on Blood and Hair Levels of Cadmium, Lead and Mercury." In: Third Conference on Vitamin C. Annals of the New York Academy of Sciences. Vol. 498.
39. Calleja, H. B., Brooks, R. H. 1960. "Acute Hepatitis Treated with High Doses of Vitamin C." *Ohio State Medical Journal*, 56:821–823.
40. Cameron, E., Campbell, A. 1974. "The Orthomolecular Treatment of Cancer." II. Clinical Trial of High-Dose Ascorbic Acid Supplements in Advanced Human Cancer. *Chemical-Biological Interactions*, 9:4, 285–315.
41. Cameron, E. 1976. "Supplemental Ascorbate in the Supportive Treatment of Cancer: Prolongation of Survival Times in Terminal Human Cancer." Proceedings of the National Academy of Sciences, 73:10, 3685–3689.
42. Cameron, E. & Pauling, L. 1978. "Supplemental Ascorbate in the Supportive Treatment of Cancer. Reevaluation of Prolongation of Survival Times in Terminal Human Cancer." *PNAS*, 75:4538–42.
43. Cameron, E. & Pauling, L. 1979. *Cancer and Vitamin C*. Linus Pauling Institute.
44. Cameron, E. 1987. "The Vitamin C and Cancer Story: A Personal Perspective." In: Nutrition, Health and

Peace. Pauling Symposia. Vol. I. Linus Pauling Institute. Jariwalla, R. J., Schwoebel, S. L. (eds).

45. Castelli, W. P. 1986. "Incidence of Coronary Heart Disease and Lipoprotein Cholesterol Levels. The Framingham Study." *JAMA*, 256: 2835–38.–1,0

46. Cathcart, R. F. 1981. "Vitamin C Titrating to Bowel Tolerance, Anascorbemia, and Acute Induced Scurvy." *Medical Hypotheses*, 7:1359–76.

47. Cathcart, R. F. 1984. "Vitamin C in the Treatment of Acquired Immune Deficiency Syndrome (AIDS)." *Medical Hypotheses*, 14:423–33.

48. Cathcart, R. F. 1988. "AIDS Treatment Using Ascorbic Acid." *Townsend Letter for Doctors.*

49. Cathcart, R. F. 1989. Letter. Personal Communication.

50. Challem, J. J. 1983. *Vitamin C Updated.* Keats Publishing.

51. Charleston, S. S. & Clegg, K. M. 1972. "Ascorbic Acid and the Common Cold." *Lancet*, 1: 1401.

52. Cheraskin, E., Ringsdorf, W. M., Jr. 1964. "Vitamin C State in a Dental School Patient Population." *Journal of the Southern California State Dental Association*, 32:10, 375–378.

53. Cheraskin, E. et al. 1968. "Effect of Diet Upon Radiation Response in Cervical Carcinoma and Uterus: A Preliminary Report." *Cryptologica*, 12:433–438.

54. Cheraskin, E., Ringsdorf,. W. M. & Sisley, E. 1983. *The Vitamin C Connection. Getting Well and Staying Well with Vitamin C.* Harper & Row.

55. Chope, H. D. & Breslow, L. 1955. "Nutritional Status of the Aging American." *Journal of Public Health*, 46: 61–7.

56. Chowka, P. B. 1988. "Cancer 1988. Is a Healing Peace in the Government's War on Cancer Finally at Hand?"

57. Cohen, A. M., Bavly, S., Poznanski, R. 1961. "Change of Diet of Yemenite Jews in Relation to Diabetes and Ischaemic Heart-Disease." *Lancet*, 2:1399–1401.

58. Cortinovis, A. et al. 1960. "Ascorbic Acid and Atherosclerosis." *Giornale di Gerontologia* (Firenze), 8:28–31.

59. Cousins, N. 1983. *The Healing Heart.* Norton.

60. Cox, M. A. 1981. *Oxycal vs. Arthritis.* Ralph Tanner Associates.

61. Creagan, et al. 1979. "Failure of High-Dose Vitamin C (Ascorbic Acid) Therapy to Benefit Patients with Advanced Cancer: A Controlled Trial." *New England Journal of Medicine*, 301:13, 687–690.
62. Dahl, H., Degre, M. 1976. "The Effect of Ascorbic Acid on Production of Human Interferon and the Antiviral Activity In Vitro." *Acta Pathologica et Microbiologica Scandinavica*, 84:5, 280–284.
63. Dainow, I. 1943. "Treatment of Herpes Zoster with Vitamin C." *Dermatologia*, 68:pp.197–201.
64. Dalton, W. L. 1962. "Massive Doses of Vitamin C in the Treatment of Viral Diseases." *Journal Indiana State Medical Association*, 55:pp.1151–1154.
65. Davies, S. & Stewart, A. 1987. *Nutritional Medicine*. Pan Books.
66. Dawson, E. B., Harris, W. A., Rankin, W. E., Charpentier, L. A., McGanity, W. J. 1987. "Effects of Ascorbic Acid on Male Fertility." In: Third Conference on Vitamin C. Annals of the New York Academy of Sciences, Vol. 498.
67. Deeniham, M. J. 1989. "Acute Oral Toxicity." Toxicology Laboratory Services, Northview Pacific Laboratories Inc.
68. Degkwitz, E. 1987. "Some Effects of Vitamin C May Be Indirect, Since It Affects the Blood Levels of Cortisol and Thyroid Hormones." In: Third Conference on Vitamin C. Annals of the New York Academy of Sciences. Vol. 498.
69. Dent, F. M. et al. 1950. *American Journal of Physiology*, 163:700.
70. Di Fabio, A. 1982. *Rheumatoid Diseases Cured at Last*. Rheumatoid Disease Foundation.
71. Di Fabio, A. 1988. *The Art of Gettting Well*. Rheumatoid Disease Foundation.
72. Diliberto, E. J., Jr., Menniti, F. S., Knoth, J., Daniels, A. J., Kizer, J. S., Viveros O. H. "Adrenomedullary Chromaffin Cells as a Model to Study the Neurobiology of Ascorbic Acid: From Monooxygenation to Neuromodulation." In: Third Conference on Vita-

min C. 1987. Annals of the New York Academy of Sciences, Vol. 498.

73. Dokter, C. E. 1983. Clinical Evaluation.

74. Erasmus, U. 1986. *Fats and Oils, the Complete Guide to Fats and Oils in Health and Nutrition.* Alive Books Publishing.

75. Erasmus, U. 1988. "Fats that Heal, Fats that Kill." Lecture. Cancer Control Society Convention.

76. Evans, W. 1938. "Vitamin C in Heart Failure." *Lancet,* 1:pp.308–309.

77. Federova, E. P. 1960. "Long-Term Ascorbic Acid Therapy for Patients with Coronary Atherosclerosis." *Sovetskaia Meditsiana* (Moskva), 25:pp.56–60.

78. Fidanza, A., Audisio, M., Mastroviacovo, P. 1982. "Vitamin C and Cholesterol" in *Vitamin C: New Clinical Applications in Immunology, Lipid Metabolism, and Cancer,* ed. A. Hanck. Hans Huber, Bern, pp.153– 171.

79. Free, V., Sanders, P. 1978. "The Use of Ascorbic Acid and Mineral Supplements in the Detoxification of Narcotic Addicts." *Journal of Orthomolecular Psychiatry,* 7:4, 264–270.

80. Furth, A. & Harding, J. 1989. "Why Sugar is Bad for You." *New Scientist,* 23 Sept., 44–7.

81. Gale, E. T., Thewlis, M. W. 1953. "Vitamin C and P in Cardiovascular and Cerebrovascular Disease." *Geriatrics,* 8:80–87.

82. Gey, K. F., Stahelin, H. B., Evans, A. "Relationship of Plasma Level of Vitamin C to Mortality from Ischemic Heart Disease." In: Third Conference on Vitamin C. 1987. Annals of the New York Academy of Sciences, Vol. 498.

83. Ginter, E. et al. 1969. "The Effect of Chronic Hypovitaminosis C on the Metabolism of Cholesterol and Atherogenesis in Guinea Pigs." *Journal of Atherosclerosis Research,* 10:341–352.

84. Ginter, E. 1973. "Cholesterol: Vitamin C Controls Its Transformation to Bile Acids." *Science,* 179:74, 702– 704.

85. Ginter, E. et al. 1977. "Effects of Ascorbic Acid on Plasma Cholesterol in Humans in a Long-Term Ex-

periment." *International Journal of Vitamin Nutrition Research*, 47(2):123–134.

86. Ginter, E. 1980. "The Role of Vitamin C in Lipid Metabolism." Presented at a symposium entitled "Vitamin C—Its Pharmacologic Activity and Nutritional Aspects," Mexico City, Mexico, National Commission of Fruiticulture.

87. Ginter, E. 1982. "Vitamin C in the Control of Hypercholesteremia in Man" in *Vitamin C: New Clinical Applications in Immunology, Lipid Metabolism, and Cancer*, ed. A. Hanck. Hans Huber, Bern, pp.137–152.

88. Ginter, E., Jurcovincova, M. "Chronic Vitamin C Deficiency Lowers Fractional Catabolic Rate of Low-Density Lipoproteins in Guinea Pigs." In: Third Conference on Vitamin C. 1987. Annals of the New York Academy of Sciences. Vol. 498.

89. Glembotski, C.C. "The Role of Ascorbic Acid in the Biosynthesis of the Neuroendocrine Peptides a-MSHd TRH." In: Third Conference on Vitamin C 1987. Annals of the New York Academy of Sciences. Vol. 498.

90. Goertz, E. 1986. "Clinical Data on Ester-C." Report on 20 Cases.

91. Graham, J. & Odent, M. 1986. *The Z. Factor. How Zinc is Vital to Your Health*. Thorsons.

92. Greer, E. 1955. "Vitamin C in Acute Poliomyelitis." *Medical Times* (Manhasset), 83:pp.1160–1161.

93. Griffith, H. W. 1988. *Complete Guide to Vitamins, Minerals & Supplements*. Fisher.

94. Gsell, O., Kalt, F. 1954. "Treatment of Epidemic Poliomyelitis with High Doses of Ascorbic Acid." *Schweizerische Medizinische Wochenschrift*, 84:661–666.

95. Haid, H. 1941. "Vitamin C in Blood in Insulin Shock." *Zeitschrift fur Klinische Medizin*, 139:p.485.

96. Hallberg, L., Brune, M., Rossander-Hulthen, L. "Is There a Physiological Role of Vitamin C in Iron Absorption?" In: Third Conference on Vitamin C. 1987. Annals of the New York Academy of Sciences. Vol. 498.

97. Harakeh, S., Jariwalla, R. J., & Pauling, L. 1990. "Suppression of human immunodeficiency virus replica-

tion by ascorbate in chronically and acutely infected cells." Proc. National Academy of Science, USA. Vol. 87pp. 724–49, Sept. 1990.

98. Harris, A., Robinson, A. B., Pauling, L. 1973. "Blood Plasma L-Ascorbic Acid Concentration for Oral L-Ascorbic Acid Dosage up to 12 Grams per Day." International Research Communications System, page 19, December.

99. Hausman, P. 1987. *The Right Dose. How to Take Vitamins & Minerals Safely.* Rodale Press.

100. Hay, L. L. 1984. *You Can Heal Your Life.* Eden Grove.

101. Heikkila, R. E., Manzino, L. "Ascorbic Acid, Redox Cycling, Lipid Peroxidation and the Binding of Dopamine Receptor Antagonists." In: Third Conference on Vitamin C. 1987. Annals of the New York Academy of Sciences. Vol. 498.

102. Herbert, V., Jacob, E. 1974. "Destruction of Vitamin B_{12} by Ascorbic Acid." *Journal of the American Medical Association*, 230:241–242.

103. Hogenkamp, H. P. C. 1980. "The Interaction Between Vitamin B_{12} and Vitamin C." *The American Journal of Clinical Nutrition*, 33:1, 1–3.

104. Holden, M., Resnick, R. J. 1936. "In Vitro Action of Synthetic Crystalline Vitamin C (Ascorbic Acid) on Herpes Virus." *Journal of Immunology*, 31:455–462.

105. Holden, M., Molloy, E. 1937. "Further Experiments on Inactivation of Herpes by Vitamin C (1-ascorbic acid)." Ibid., 33:251–257.

106. Hornig, G., Weiser, H., Weber, F. & Wiss, O. 1973. "Effect of Massive Doses of Ascorbic Acid on its Catabolism in Guinea Pigs." *Inter. J. Vit. & Nutrition Res.* 43(1) 28–33.

107. Hornig, D. "Recent advances in Vitamin C Metabolism. 1974. In: Second Conference on Vitamin C." Annals of the New York Academy of Science, 91–103.

108. Horrobin, D. F., Manku, M. S., Oka, M., Morgan, R. O., Cunnane, S. C., Ally, A. I., Ghayur, T., Schweitzer, M., Karmaki, R. A. 1979. "The Nutritional Regulation of T Lymphocyte Function." *Medical Hypotheses*, 5:969–985.

109. Horrobin, D. F., Oka, M., Manku, M. S. 1979. "The Regulation of Prostaglandin E Formation: A Candidate for One of the Fundamental Mechanisms Involved in the Actions of Vitamin C. *Medical Hypotheses*, 5:849–858.

110. Houston, R. G. 1987. Repression and Reform in the Evaluation of Alternative Cancer Therapies.

111. Hume & Weyers, E. 1973. "Changes in Leucocyte Ascorbic Acid During the Common Cold." *Scottish Medical Journal*, 18:3–7.

112. Ibric, L. L. V., Sevanian, A. Effects of Ascorbic and Dehydroascorbic Acids on Lipid Composition of C_3 H/10T$^{1/2}$ Cells. In: Third Conference on Vitamin C. 1987. Annals of the New York Academy of Sciences. Vol. 498.

113. Jacob, R. A., Omaye, S. T., Skala, J. H., Leggott, P. J., Rothman, D. L., Murray, P. A. "Experimental Vitamin C Depletion and Supplementation in Young Men." In: Third Conference on Vitamin C. 1987. Annals of the New York Academy of Sciences. Vol. 498.

114. Jaffe, R. M., Kasten, B., Young, D. S., MacLowry, J. D. 1975. "False-Negative Stool Occult Blood Tests Caused by Ingestion of Ascorbic Acid (Vitamin C)." *Annals of Internal Medicine*, 83:6, 824–826.

115. Jaffe, R. M., Lawrence, L., Schmid, A., MacLowry, J. D. 1979. "Inhibition by Ascorbic Acid (Vitamin C) of Chemical Detection of Blood in Urine." *American Journal of Clinical Pathology*, 72:3, 468–470.

116. Jaffe, R. M., Zierdt, W. 1979. "A New Occult Blood Test Not Subject to False-Negative Results from Reducing Substances." *Journal of Laboratory and Clinical Medicine*, 93:5, 879–886.

117. Jariwalla, R. J., Schwoebel, S. L. (eds). 1987. Nutrition, Health and Peace. Pauling Symposia. Vol. I. Linus Pauling Institute.

118. Johnson, G. E., Obenshain, S. S. 1981. "Nonresponsiveness of Serum High-Density Lipoprotein-Cholesterol to High Dose Ascorbic Acid Administration in Normal Men." *American Journal of Clinical Nutrition*, 34:2088–2091.

119. Jungeblut, C. W. 1935. "Inactivation of Poliomyelitis Virus by Crystallin Vitamin C (Ascorbic Acid)." *Journal of Experimental Medicine*, 62:517–521.

120. Jungeblut, C. W. 1939. "Further Observations on Vitamin C Therapy in Experimental Poliomyelitis." *Journal of Experimental Medicine*, 65:127–146. 1937. Ibid., 66:459–477, 1937. Ibid., 70:315–332.

121. Jungeblut, C. W. 1939. "A Further Contribution to the Vitamin C Therapy in Experimental Poliomyelitis." *Journal of Experimental Medicine*, 70:327.

122. Kallner, A. "Requirement for Vitamin C Based on Metabolic Studies." In: Third Conference on Vitamin C. 1987. Annals of the New York Academy of Sciences. Vol. 498.

123. Kapeghian, J. C. & Verlangieri, A. J. 1984. "The Effects of Glucose on Ascorbic Acid Uptake in Heart Endothelial Cells: Possible Pathogenesis of Diabetic Angiopathies." *Life Sciences*, 34: 577–84.

124. Katz, S. M., DiSilvio, T. V. 1973. "Ascorbic Acid Effects on Serum Glucose Values." *Journal of the American Medical Association*, 224:5, 628.

125. Kirchmair, H. 1957. "Treatment of Epidemic Hepatitis in Children with High Doses of Ascorbic Acid." *Medizinische Monatschrift*, 11:353–357. 1957. "Epidemic Hepatitis in Children." *Deutsche Gesundheitwesen*, 12:pp.773–774. 1957. "Epidemic Hepatitis in Children and Its Treatment with High Doses of Ascorbic Acid." Ibid., 12:1525–1536. 1957.

126. Klenner, F. R. 1948. "Virus Pneumonia and Its Treatment with Vitamin C." *Southern Medicine and Surgery*, 110:34–36.

127. Klenner, F. R. "The Treatment of Poliomyelitis and Other Virus Diseases with Vitamin C." *Southern Medicine and Surgery*, 111:209–214. 1949. "Massive Doses of Vitamin C and the Virus Diseases." Ibid., 113: 101–107. 1951. "The Vitamin and Massage Treatment for Acute Poliomyelitis." Ibid., 114:194–197. 1952. "The Use of Vitamin C as an Antibiotic." *Journal of Applied Nutrition*, 6: 274–278. 1953. "The Folly in the Continued Use of a Killed Polio Virus Vaccine." *Tri-State Medical Journal*, Feb. 1959:1–8.

128. Klenner, F. R. 1951. "Massive Doses of Vitamin C and the Viral Diseases." *Southern Medicine and Surgery*, 113:101–107.

129. Klenner, F. R. 1971. "Observations on the Dose and Administration of Ascorbic Acid When Employed Beyond the Range of a Vitamin in Human Pathology." *Journal of Applied Nutrition*, 23:3–4, 61–88.

130. Kligler, I. J., Bernkopf, H. 1937. "Inactivation of Vaccinia Virus by Ascorbic Acid and Glutathione." *Nature* 139:965–966.

131. Kolmakov, V. N. 1957. "Effect of Vitamin C on Hypercholesterolmia in Fasting Rabbits." *Voprosy Meditsinskoi Khimii* (Moskva), 3:414–419.

132. Lamden, M. P., Chrystowski, G. A. 1954. "Urinary Oxalate Excretion by Man Following Ascorbic Acid Ingestion." Proceedings of the Society for Experimental Biology and Medicine 85:190–192.

133. Langenbusch, W., Enderling, A. 1937. "Einfluss der Vitamine auf das Virus der Maul-und Klavenseuch." *Zentralblatt fur Bakteriologie*, 140:112–115.

134. Lee W., Davis K. A., Rettmer, L. R., Labbe, R. F. 1988. "Ascorbic Acid Status: Biochemical and Clinical Considerations." *Am. J. Clin. Nutr.* 48: 286–90.

135. Leibovitz, B. 1984. *Carnitine: The Vitamin B_T Phenomenon.* Dell, New York.

136. Levine, M. & Morita K. 1985. "Ascorbic Acid in Endocrine systems." In: *Vitamins and Hormones*. Vol. 42. Academic Press.

137. Levine, M., Morita K., Heldman & Pollard H. B. 1985. "Ascorbic Acid Regulation of Norephinephrine Biosynthesis in Isolated Chromaffin Granules from Bovine Adrenal Medulla." *J. Biol. Chem.* 260 (29): 15598–15603.

138. Levine, M. 1986. "New Concepts in the Biology and Biochemistry of Ascorbic Acid." *The New England Journal of Medicine*, 314:14, 892–902.

139. Levine, M. 1986. "Ascorbic Acid Specifically Enhances Dopamine Monoxygenease Activity in Resting and Stimulated Chromaffin Cells." *J. Biol. Chem.*, 261(16): 7347–56.

Bibliography

140. Levin, M., Hartzell, W. 1987. "Ascorbic Acid: The Concept of Optimum Requirements." In: Third Conference on Vitamin C. 1987. Annals of The New York Academy of Sciences. Vol. 498.

141. Lohmann, W. "Ascorbic Acid and Cataract; Varma, S. D. Ascorbic Acid and the Eye with Special Reference to the Lens." In: Third Conference on Vitamin C. 1987. Annals of the New York Academy of Sciences. vol. 498; 1989. "Vitamin C, E Supplements May Help Prevent Cataracts in Elderly." *Ophthalmology Times* Nov. 1, p. 9.

142. Lojkin, M. 1936. Contributions of the Boyce Thompson Institute, Vol. 8, No.4. L. F. Martin. Proceedings Third International Congress of Microbiology, New York, 1940, p. 281.

143. Lominski, I. 1936. "Inactivation du bacteriophage par l'acide ascorbique." *Comptes Rendus des Séances de la Société de biologie et de ses Filliales* (Paris), Vol. 122: 766–768.

144. Marcus, M., Prabhudesai, M., Wassef, S. 1980. "Stability of Vitamin B_{12} in the Presence of Ascorbic Acid in Food and Serum: Restoration by Cyanide of Apparent Loss." *The American Journal of Clinical Nutrition* 33:137–143.

145. Marcus, M. 1981. "Vitamin B_{12}: Response to Dr. Herbert." *The American Journal of Clinical Nutrition*, 34: 1622–1624.

146. Markham,. R. G. 1989. Compositions and Methods for Administering Vitamin C. United States Patent No. 4,822,816.

147. Martin, S. & Chaitow, L. 1988. *A World Without AIDS.* Thorsons.

148. Mayson, J. S., Schumaker, O., Nakamura, R. M. 1972. "False-Negative Tests for Urinary Glucose in the Presence of Ascorbic Acid." *American Journal of Clinical Pathology*, 58:3, 297–299.

149. McCormick, W. J. 1957. "Coronary Thrombosis. A New Concept of Mechanism and Etiology." *Clinical Medicine*, pp.839–845.

150. Melethil, S., Subrahmanyam, M. B., Chang, C. J., Mason, W. D. "Megadoses of Vitamin C: A Pharmacoki-

netic Evaluation." In: Third Conference on Vitamin C. 1987. Annals of the New York Academy of Sciences. Vol. 498.
151. Menten. M. L., King, C. G. 1935. "The Influence of Vitamin C Level upon Resistance to Diphtheria Toxin." *Journal of Nutrition*, 10:141–153.
152. Milner, J. E. 1980. "Ascorbic Acid in the Prevention of Chromium Dermatitis." *Journal of Occupational Medicine*, 22:1, 51–52.
153. Moertel, C. G., Fleming, T. R., Creagan, E. T., Rubin J., O'Connell, M. J., Ames, M. M. 1985. "High-Dose Vitamin C versus Placebo in the Treatment of Patients with Advanced Cancer Who Had No Prior Chemotherapy." *New England Journal of Medicine*, 312:137–141.
154. Morishige, F., Murata, A. 1978. "Prolongation of Survival Times in Terminal Human Cancer by Administration of Supplemental Ascorbate." *Journal of the International Academy of Preventive Medicine*, 5:1, 47–52.
155. Morishige, F., Murata A. 1978. "Vitamin C for Prophylaxis of Viral Hepatitis B in Transfused Patients." *Journal of the International Academy of Preventive Medicine*, 5:54–58.
156. Mueller, L. 1989. "Dysplasia's End." *Outdoor Life*. April.
157. Mumma, R. O. 1968. "Ascorbic Acid as a Sulfating Agent." *Biochimicia et Biophysica Acta*, 165:571– 573. Mumma, R. O., Verlangieri, A. J. 1971. "In Vivo Sulfation of Cholesterol by Ascorbic Acid 3-Sulfate as a Possible Explanation for the Hypocholestemic Effects of Ascorbic Acid." *Federation Proceedings*, 30:2.
158. Murata, A. 1975. "Virucidal Activity of Vitamin C: Vitamin C for Prevention and Treatment of Viral Diseases." Proceedings of the First Intersectional Congress of Microbiological Societies, Science Council of Japan, 3:432–442.
159. Nahata, M. C., McLeod. 1978. "Noneffect of Oral Ascorbic Acid on Urinary Copper Reduction Glucose Test." *Diabetes Care*, 1:1, 34–35.

Bibliography

160. Newmark, H. L., 1976. "Stability of Vitamin B_{12} in the Presence of Ascorbic Acid." *American Journal of Clinical Nutrition*, 29:6, 645–649.

161. Niki, E. "Interaction of Ascorbate and a-Tocopherol." In: Third Conference on Vitamin C. 1987. Annals of the New York Academy of Sciences. Vol. 498.

162. Omaye, S. T., Schaus, E. E., Kutnink, M. A., Hawkes, W. C. "Measurement of Vitamin C in Blood Components by High-Performance Liquid Chromatography: Implication in Assessing Vitamin C Status." In: Third Conference on Vitamin C. 1987. Annals of the New York Academy of Sciences. Vol. 498.

163. Paez de la Torre, J. M. 1945. "Ascorbic Acid in Measles." *Archives Argentinos do Pediatria*, 24:225–227.
     Paterson, J. C. 1941. "Some Factors in the Causation of Intimal Hemorrhages and in the Precipitation of Coronary Thrombi." *Canadian Medical Association Journal*, 44:114–120.

164. Pauling, L. 1970. *Vitamin C the Common Cold and the Flu.* Berkley.

165. Pauling, L. et al. 1985. "Effect of Ascorbic Acid on the Incidence of Spontaneous Mammary Tumors in RIII Mice." *PNAS* 82:5185–89.

166. Pauling, L. 1986. *How to Live Longer and Feel Better.* Avon Books.

167. Pecoraro, R. E., Chen, M. S. "Ascorbic Acid Metabolism in Diabetes Mellitus." In: Third Conference on Vitamin C. 1987. Annals of the New York Academy of Sciences. Vol. 498.

168. Pfeiffer, C. C. 1987. "Mental Illness and Schizophrenia." *The Nutrition Connection.* Thorsons.

169. Pfleger, R., Scholl, F. 1937. "Diabetes and Vitamin C." *Wiener Archiv fur Innere Medizin*, 31:pp.219–229.

170. Prauer, H. W. 1971. "Vitamin C and Tests for Diabetes." *New England Journal of Medicine*, 284:23, 1328.

171. Prinz, Wetal. 1977. "The Effect of Ascorbic Acid Supplementation on Some Parameters of Human Immunological Defence System." *Int. J. Vit. & Nut. Research*, 47: 248–56.

172. Project Cure Center for Alternative Cancer Research.

2020 K Street, NW, Suite 350, Washington DC 20069. (202) 293–3479.

173. Richards, R. K., Kueter, D., Klatt, T. J. 1941. "Effect of Vitamin C deficiency on Different Types of Barbiturates." *Proc. Soc. Exp. Biol. Med.*, 48: 403–9.

174. Rineheart, J. F., Mettier, S. R. 1934. "The Heart Valves and Muscle in Experimental Scurvy with Superimposed Infection." *American Journal of Pathology*, 10: 61–79.

175. Ringsdorf, W. M., Jr., Cheraskin, E. 1978. "Lingual Ascorbic Acid Test." *Quintessence International*, 12:1707, 81–85.

176. Ringsdorf, W. M., Jr., Cheraskin, E. 1979. "Vitamin C and the Metabolism of Analgesic, Antipyretic, and Anti-Inflammatory Drugs: A Review." *Alabama Journal of Medical Sciences*, 16:3, 217–220.

177. Ringsdorf, W. M., Jr., Cheraskin, E. 1982. "Vitamin C and Human Wound Healing." *Oral Surgery*, 53:231–236.

178. Rivers, J. M. "Safety of High-level Vitamin C Ingestion." In: Third Conference on Vitamin C. 1987. Annals of the New York Academy of Sciences. Vol. 498.

179. *Recommended Dietary Allowances.* National Academy of Sciences. Washington. Nat. Acad. Press 1980, p.75.

180. Rogoff, J. M. et al. 1944. "Vitamin C and Insulin Action." *Pennsylvania Medical Journal*, 47:579–582.

181. Romney, S. L., Basu, J., Vermund, S., Palen, P. R., Duttagupta, C. "Plasma Reduced and Total Ascorbic Acid in Human Uterine Cervix Dysplasias and Cancer." In: Third Conference on Vitamin C. 1987. Annals of the New York Academy of Sciences. Vol. 498.

182. Rose, R. C. "Ascorbic Acid Protection Against Free Radicals." In: Third Conference on Vitamin C. 1987. Annals of the New York Academy of Sciences. Vol. 498.

183. Rossander, L., Hallberg, L., Bjorn-Rasmussen, E. 1979. "Absorption of Iron from Breakfast Meals." *American Journal of Clinical Nutrition*, 32:12, 2484–2489.

184. Ruskin, S. L. 1952. Crystalline Calcium Ascorbate and Methods of Preparing Same. United States Patent Office No. 2,596,103.

185. Sabin, A. B. 1939. "Vitamin C in Relation to Experimental Poliomyelitis." *Journal of Experimental Medicine*, 69:507–515.

186. Samitz, M. H. 1970. "Ascorbic Acid in the Prevention and Treatment of Toxic Effects of Chromates." *Acta Dermatovenereologica* 50:1, 59–64.

187. Scher, J., et al. 1976. "Massive Vitamin C as an Adjunct in Methadone Maintenance and Detoxification of Narcotic Addicts." *Journal of Orthomolecular Psychiatry*, 5:3, 191–198.

188. Schmidt, Karl-Heinz et al. 1981. "Urinary Oxalate Excretion After Large Intakes of Ascorbic Acid in Man." *The American Journal of Clinical Nutrition*, 34:305–311.

189. Sebrov, K. R. 1956. "Prophylaxis and Treatment of Arteriosclerosis with Ascorbic Acid." *Terapevticheskii Arkhiv* (Moskva), 28:55–65.

190. Shaffer, C. F. 1970. "Ascorbic Acid and Atherosclerosis." *American Journal of Clinical Nutrition*, 23:27–30.

191. Sigal, A., King C. G. 1936. "The Relationship of Vitamin C to Glucose Tolerance in the Guinea Pig." *Journal of Biological Chemistry*, 116:489–492.

192. Smith, J. L., Hodges, R. E. "Serum Levels of Vitamin C in Relation to Dietary and Supplemental Intake of Vitamin C in Smokers and Nonsmokers." In: Third Conference on Vitamin C. 1987. Annals of the New York Academy of Sciences. Vol. 498.

193. Sokoloff, B. et al. 1967. "Effect of Ascorbic Acid on Certain Blood Fat Metabolism Factors in Animals and Man." *Journal of Nutrition*, 91:107–118.

194. Spiegel, H. E. & Pinili, E. 1974. "Effect of Vitamin C on SGOT, SGPT, LDH & Bilirubin." *Med. J. of Australia* 2(7) 265–6.

195. Spittle, C. R. 1971. "Atherosclerosis and Vitamin C." *Lancet*, 2:1280–1281.

196. Spittle, C. R. 1974. "The Action of Vitamin C on Blood Vessels." *American Heart Journal*, 88:3, 387–388.

197. Stahelin, H. B., Gey K. F., Brubacher, G. "Plasma Vitamin C and Cancer Death: The Prospective Basel Study." In: Third Conference on Vitamin C. 1987. Annals of the New York Academy of Sciences. Vol. 498.

198. Stewart, C. T. et al. 1952. "Factors Determining Effect of Insulin on Metabolism of Glucose in Ascorbic Acid Deficiency and Scurvy in the Monkey." *American Journal of Diseases of Children*, 84:677–690.
199. Stone, I. 1965. "Studies of a Mammalian Enzyme System for Producing Evolutionary Evidence on Man." *Amer. J. Physical Anthrop.*, 23: 83–86.
200. Stone, I. 1972. *The Healing Factor: Vitamin C against Disease.* Grosset & Dunlap.
201. Stone, N., Meister, A. 1962. "Function of Ascorbic Acid in the Conversion of the Proline to Collagen Hydroxyproline." *Nature*, 194:555.
202. Szent-Györgyi, A. 1937. "Studies on Biological Oxidation and Some of Its Catalysts." Szeged, Hungary.
203. Tajima, S., Pinnell, S. R. 1982. "Regulations of Collagen Synthesis by Ascorbic Acid: Ascorbic Acid Increases Type I Procollagen mRNA." *Biochemical and Biophysical Research Communications*, 106:632–637.
204. Tannenbaum, S. T., Wishnok, J. S. "Inhibition of Nitrosamine Formation by Ascorbic Acid." In: Third Conference on Vitamin C. 1987. Annals of the New York Academy of Sciences. Vol. 498.
205. Taylor, S. 1937. "Scurvy and Carditis." *Lancet*, 1:973–979.
206. Thomas, C. B., Holljes, H. W. D., Eisenberg, F. F. 1961. "Observations on Seasonal Variations in Total Serum Cholesterol Level Among Healthy Young Prisoners." *Annals of Internal Medicine*, 54:3, 413–430.
207. Thomas, M., Hughes, R. E. 1985. "Evaluation of Threonic Acid Toxicity in Small Animals." *Food Chemistry*, 17:79–83.
208. Thomas, W. R., Holt, R. G. 1978. "Vitamin C and Immunity: An Assessment of the Evidence." *Clinical Experimental Immunology*, 32:370–379.
209. Tiapina, L. A. 1961. "The Effect of Ascorbic Acid on Blood Lipids in Essential Hypertension and Atherosclerosis." *Cor et Vasa* (Praha), 3:98–106.
210. Trang, J. M., Blanchard, J., 1982. "The Effect of Vitamin C on the Pharmacokinetics of Caffeine in Elderly Men." *Amer. J. Clin. Nutri.*, 35:487–94.

Bibliography

211. Trimmer, R. W., Lundy, C. J. 1948. "A Nutrition Survey in Heart Disease." *American Practitioner*, Vol. 2: 448–450.
212. Tsao, C. S. and Salimi, S. L., Pauling, L. 1982. "Lack of Effect of Ascorbic Acid on Calcium Excretion." *IRCS Medical Science*, 10:738.
213. Tsao, C. S. and Salimi, S. L. (1984) "Effects of Large Intake of Ascorbic Acid on Urinary and Plasma Oxalic Acid Levels." *International Journal of Nutrition and Vitamin Research*, 54:245–249.
214. Tsao, C. S. and Salimi, S. L. 1984. "Evidence of Rebound Effect with Ascorbic Acid." *Medical Hypotheses*, 13:303–310.
215. Turley, S. D., West, C. E., Horton, B. J. 1976. "The Role of Ascorbic Acid in the Regulation of Cholesterol Metabolism and in the Pathogenesis of Atherosclerosis." *Atherosclerosis*, 24:1–18.
216. Uverskaia, V. T. 1958. "Influence of Ascorbic Acid on Cholesterolemia and Acid-Base Balance in Patients with Hypertensive Disease and Atherosclerosis." *Trudy Leningradskogo Sanitarnogigienicheskogo Meditsinskego Instituta*, 40: 150–158.
217. Vallance, S. (1977). "Relationships between Ascorbic Acid and Serum Proteins of the Immune System." *British Medical Journal*, 2: 437–438.
218. Vargus, Magne R. 1963. "Vitamin C in Treatment of Influenza." *El Dia Medico*, Vol.35:1714–1715.
219. Verlangieri, A. J. 1973. "Possible Biological & Pharmacological Significance of L-Ascorbic Acid & L-Ascorbic Acid 2-Sulphate on Cholesterol Metabolism, Metabolic Sulfation and Atherogenesis." Ph.D. Thesis. Penn. State Univ.
220. Verlangieri, A. J. and Stevens, J. W. 1979. L-Ascorbic Acid: Effects on Aortic Glycosaminoglycan ^{35}S Incorporation in Rabbit Induced Atherogenesis Blood Vessels. 16(4):177–85.
221. Verlangieri, A. J. & Sestito, J. 1981. "Effect of Insulin on Ascorbic Acid Uptake by Heart Endothelial Cells: Possible Relationship to Retinal Atherogeneses." *Life Sciences*, 29:5–9.

222. Verlangieri, A. J., Bush, M. J. and Kapeghian. 1984. "Duplex Ultrasound Analysis of the Carotid Arteries in Macaca Fascicularis." *J. Card. Ultrason.*, 2 (4): 293–302.
223. Verlangieri, A. J. 1985. "The Role of Vitamin C in Diabetic and Nondiabetic Atherosclerosis." Bulletin, Bureau of Pharm. Services, Univ. Miss. Vol. 21.
224. Verlangieri, A. J., Cardin, B. A. and Bush, M. 1985. "The Interaction of Aortic Glycosaminoglycans and ^{3}-Insulin Endothelial Permeability in Cholesterol Induced Rabbit Atherogenesis."
225. Verlangieri, A. J. 1987. "Acute Study to Determine the Relative Gastro-Intestinal Absorption of Ester-C^R, as Compared to L-Ascorbic Acid."
226. Verlangieri, A. J. 1988. "Acute Study to Determine the Relative Rate of Absorption and Excretion of Ester-C Calcium Ascorbate, USP Calcium Ascorbate with an added Metabolite and 'Another Commercial Ascorbate.' "
227. Verlangieri, A. J. "Acute Study to determine the Relative Rate of Absorption and Excretion of Ester-C^R, Calcium Ascorbate, and Calcium Threonate and Renatured Vitamin C."
228. Verlangieri, A. J. 1988. "Acute Study to Determine the Relative Rate of Absorption and Excretion of USP Calcium Ascorbate and Ester-C Calcium Ascorbate."
229. Verlangieri, A. J. 1989. "The Effects of Calcium-L-Threonate, Calcium Lyxonate, Calcium Xylonate and Threonolactone on the Uptake of ^{14}C-L-Ascorbic Acid into 3T3 Mouse Fibroblasts in Culture."
230. Verlangieri, A. J. 1989. "Effects of Vitamin C and Vitamin E on Induced Primate Atherosclerosis." Manuscript submitted.
231. Wapnick, A. A. 1969. "The Effect of Ascorbic Acid Deficiency on Desferrioxamine-Induced Urinary Iron Excretion." *British Journal of Haematology*, 17:6, 563–568.
232. Wassertheil-Smoller, S. 1981. "Dietary Vitamin C and Uterine Cervical Dysplasia." *American Journal of Epidemiology*, 114:5, 714–724.

Bibliography

233. Waugh, W. A., King, C. G. 1932. Isolation and Identification of Vitamin C. *Journal of Biological Chemistry*, 97:325–331.

234. Werbach, M. R. 1987. *Nutritional Influences on Illness.* Thorsons, Keats Publishing.

235. Willis, G. C. 1953. "An Experimental Study of the Intimal Hermorrhages and in the Precipitation of Coronary Thrombi." *Canadian Medical Association Journal*, 69:17–22.

236. Willis, G. C. et al. 1954. "Serial Arteriography in Atherosclerosis." *Canadian Medical Association Journal*, 71:562–568.

237. Willis, G. C., Fishman, S. 1955. "Ascorbic Acid Content of Human Arterial Tissue." *Canadian Medical Association Journal*, 72:500–503.

238. Willis, G. C. 1957. "The Influence of Ascorbic Acid upon the Liver." *Canadian Medical Association Journal*, 76:1044–1048.

239. Willis, G. C. 1957. "The Reversibility of Atherosclerosis." Canadian Medical Association *Journal of Nutrition*, 77:106–109.

240. Wilson, P. W., Garrison, R. J. 1980. "Prevalence of Coronary Heart Disease in the Framingham Offspring Study: Role of Lipoprotein Cholesterol." *Am. J. Cardiol.*, 46: 649–54.

241. Wright, J. V. and Suen, R. M. 1987. "A Clinical Study of Ester-C vs L-Ascorbic Acid." Meridian Valley Clinical Laboratory.

242. Yonemoto, R. H., Chretien, P. B., Fehniger, T. F. 1976. "Enhanced Lymphocyte Blastogenesis by Oral Ascorbic Acid." Proceedings of the American Association for Cancer Research 17:288.

243. Yudkin,. J., Edelman, I., Hough, L., (Eds.) 1971. *Sugar: Chemical Biological, and Nutritional Aspects of Sucrose.* Daniel Davey, Hartford, Conn.

244. Yudkin, J. 1972. *Sweet and Dangerous.* Peter H. Wyden, New York.

245. Zannoni, V. G., Brodfuehrer, J. I., Smart, R. C., Susick R. L., Jr. "Ascorbic Acid, Alcohol, and Environmental Chemicals." In: Third Conference on Vitamin C.

1987. Annals of the New York Academy of Sciences. Vol. 498.

246. Zureick, M. 1950. "Treatment of Shingles and Herpes with Vitamin C Intravenously." *Journal des Praticiens*, 64:586.

INDEX

167

Metabolites,
definition of, 34–35
effect on acquired immunodeficiency syndrome
(AIDS), 83–90
function of, 101–103
vitamin C and, 97–98
Methadone, interaction of
vitamin C with, 29
Methotrexate, as anti-arthritic
drug, 64
Mettier, S.R., 51, 55
Minerals,
as dietary supplement, 119
vitamin C interaction and,
27–31
zinc interaction with vitamin, C, 28
Moertel, C.G., 75
Mononucleosis, therapeutic
use of vitamin C for,
11
Morgan, R.O., 39
Morishige, F., 73
Morita, K., 98
Mueller, L., 69
Mumma, R.O., 56
Murata, A., 56, 73, 98

Nahata, M.C., 25, 56
National Academy of Sci-
ences, 3, 104
National Institutes of Health
(NIH), view on vitamin
C/AIDS relationship, 89
Neurotransmitter synthesis,
functional metabolic
rates of vitamin, C, 98
New York Academy of Sci-
ence Conference on
Vitamin, C, 43
Newmark, H.L., 22–23
Niki, E., 43–46, 98

Non-steroidal anti-inflammatory
agents (NSAIDS), as anti-
arthritic drug, 63
Nuclear magnetic response
(NMR) spectroscopy,
High pressure liquid
chromatography
(HPLC) and, 94

Obenshain, S.S., 130
O'Connell, M.J., 75
Oka, M., 39, 42, 98
Omaye, S.T., 111
Oral drugs, interaction of
vitamin C with, 29
Oxygen-hemoglobin, modula-
tor of dissociation curve,
98

Paez de la Torre, J.M., 55
Pain, therapeutic use of vita-
min C for, 11
Palen, P.R., 73, 76
Paterson, J.C., 55
Pauling, L., 5–6, 20–23, 26,
38, 41, 49–54, 72–75,
78–80, 98, 106, 114,
121–122
Pecoraro, R.E., 49, 60, 98
Penicillamine, as antiarthritic
drug, 63–64
Periodontal disease, therapeutic
use of vitamin C for,
11
Pfleger, R., 60
PGE1, vitamin C and, 42
PGE2, vitamin C and, 42
PGF2, vitamin C and, 42
Pinili, E., 25, 56
Pinnell, S.R., 57
Poliomyelitis, disease of, 4
Pollard, H.B., 98

173